Hope to be Healed

Emile

Be Blessed

Love,

Karen

KAREN S. WALTHER

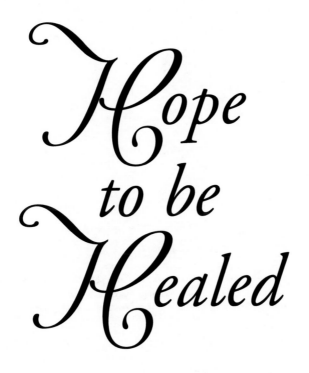

Hope
to be
Healed

Living Through Illness
& Life's Challenges

TATE PUBLISHING & *Enterprises*

Published by Tate Publishing & Enterprises, LLC
127 E. Trade Center Terrace | Mustang, Oklahoma 73064 USA
1.888.361.9473 | www.tatepublishing.com

Tate Publishing is committed to excellence in the publishing industry. The company reflects the philosophy established by the founders, based on Psalm 68:11,
"The Lord gave the word and great was the company of those who published it."

Book design copyright © 2010 by Tate Publishing, LLC. All rights reserved.
Cover design by Amber Gulilat
Interior design by Nathan Harmony

Published in the United States of America

ISBN: 978-1-61663-320-2
Religion: Christian Life: Inspirational
10.05.26

Dedication

With special thanks to our son, Dylan, who was six years old when I became ill. Even at this young age, he was my most positive encouragement and a rock for me, never complaining about carrying groceries, taking carts back to the stores, carrying laundry up and down stairs, vacuuming the house, cleaning the bathroom, and daily walking down the driveway to get the mail. He is the reason I can function in my home. I thank the Lord for such a compassionate child. I feel greatly blessed. Thank you, Dylan. I love you.

I also want to thank my family—my parents Ted and Barbara Specchio, my sister, Laura DeNardo, and my brother, Larry Specchio. They all helped me both financially and physically. I love you all for making my time on disability bearable, especially those times when money was in such short supply.

To my family and friends, you can now read about my faith and the hope that kept me going from day to day.

Acknowledgments

This book would not have made it to the press without the vision from my Lord, Jesus Christ. In addition, I am grateful for the advice, support, positive encouragement, and guidance from the following friends. I express my heartfelt admiration, appreciation, and thanks to each of them.

Susan Michael

Margaret (Margie) Levack

Sylvia J. Levey Stansfield

Mary Laurey

Judy Janowski

Cynthia Woodward

Pastor Jerry and Jean Bricker

In Appreciation

I want to thank Pastor Joseph Zaino. He was my Pastor for seven of the eight years while I wrote this book. His teaching is very "deep" and is reflected in much of my writing. Pastor Zaino is a walking/talking bible that instilled in me the truth about the Word of God. He did not sugar coat the Word and is an awesome teacher. Thank you Pastor for all the wisdom. We miss you but thank God for the time you were our Pastor. Pastor Zaino is now a Senior Pastor at a church in Tyler, Texas.

Table of Contents

Be strong and take heart,
All you who hope in the Lord.

Psalm 31:24

That Hopeless Feeling

Have you ever felt so discouraged, frightened, and hopeless when you have been diagnosed with a disease or illness? The doctors offer no hope or positive encouragement. They offer medicine, which often does not cure the illness and many times can make you worse. You live in fear of getting worse and even the fear of death.

I have discovered the secret to victory over sickness. I have met the great physician and the one who has positive promises for healing that will come to pass. "Be strong and take heart, all you who hope in the Lord" (Psalm 31:24). This scripture is the basis for my hope.

Let me take you on the journey that I am traveling and that has changed my life. How badly do you want your life to be transformed into a marvelous, healthy journey? It does not matter what you are facing. It could be multiple sclerosis, cancer, lupus, diabetes, depression, chronic fatigue, panic attacks, heart disease, stress and/or any other diseases common to man.

One of the first things I learned, and I must say the greatest, is that sickness is not from God; he is the healer: "I am the Lord who heals you" (Exodus 15:26). His Son, Jesus, died on a cross over 2,000 years ago for our sins and our sicknesses. He took whatever sickness you may be dealing with today. All you have to do is receive what he did for all of us on the cross. I know the thoughts of many of you. *I have done this or that wrong over the years, and I am being punished.* Wrong! *If only I could have been a better person, this would not have happened.* Good news! God does not make us sick to punish us. If you turn your life over to God, He he is in control and takes over. In Isaiah, God's Word says, "I am the Lord your God who teaches you what is best for you, who directs you in the way you should go" (Isaiah 48:17). He will take the sickness or whatever you may be facing and turn it around for your good. Romans 8:28 states, "And we know that in all things God works for the good of those who love him." He is a good God and wants you whole more than you want to be well. Just as we as parents want the best and will do anything for our children, he is longing to do his perfect will for you.

As I share my testimony and struggle with multiple sclerosis, I pray you will be open to receive all I share to turn your life and health around. You see, God created each one of us. Until you come to him, your life will not be complete. You will have a void, as I did, that cannot be filled with earthly desires—work, friends, and activities, even your marriage or children. Our lives here on earth are a blink of an eye compared to eternity. So much time and effort are placed on the here and now—worldly desires. You want to live on earth healthy, but where will you spend eternity? I will explain further in this book regarding my journey and the key to victory over sickness while walking in God's perfect will. Will you be a willing vessel? I have lived on both sides, and trust me, there is life and health with God at the helm of your life. My old life is a distant memory, as it was empty and full of sin and sickness. With God, old things have passed away. Behold all things become new. In 2 Corinthians 5:17, God's Word says, "If anyone is in Christ, he is a new creation; the old has gone, the new has come."

My Diagnosis

It was the fall of 1990; I was working full-time as a secretary for a local manufacturing company. It was a busy time; Jeff and I were engaged to be married. I was very active; some might have described me as hyper. I never had time or made the time to stop and enjoy life's simple pleasures. I think back now and realize how fortunate I was. If only I could do it over again, I would thank God and appreciate every step.

Our engagement was a surprise on Valentine's Day 1989 in the Cayman Islands. Although Jeff was quick to ask me to marry him, he did not want to commit to a wedding date. At that time, Jeff owned and operated a gasoline service station that was across the street from where I worked. We used to travel twice each year—in February to the islands and in May to Florida. Some may have thought life was great for us. I know now I did not appreciate my health on those trips. Now I think about the ocean, the sunsets, and walking on the beach. At the time,

I did realize the beauty; however, I did take my health for granted, as many of us do until it becomes a challenge.

In the fall of 1990, I began having tingling down both my legs. This was aggravated when I would walk fast. I noticed it especially when I walked from the office where I worked to my car. At this time I didn't experience other MS symptoms. Only now do I realize how blessed I was. The local doctors were booked for the next month, and I wanted answers as soon as possible. I was able to get an appointment within a couple of weeks with a neurologist at a clinic half an hour away from our home. Jeff was very supportive and took me to my appointments even though we were not married yet. Dr. Richard Flynn, chief of neurology at Guthrie Clinic in Sayre, Pennsylvania, told me he thought I had a mild form of MS. Wanting to have a final determination, I submitted to a spinal tap. In 1990, MRIs were not yet used for the diagnosis of MS as they are today. My spinal tap was interesting. I had to lie flat for a time afterward to avoid getting a bad headache. I laid flat as Jeff drove me home. When I went for my follow-up appointment, the spinal tap results confirmed what Dr. Flynn had suspected. I found out I had a mild form of MS, but I was pleased to hear him say I might never have to see him again. He said the tingling feelings in my legs would disappear, and he was right.

Finding out I had MS was, of course, a shock. I lived with a fear that I would wake up someday not able to walk or get out of bed. I truly did not even know what multiple sclerosis was. Upon telling the news to my parents, they of course were concerned and wanted to build a ramp into their house. I thought, *I do not need a ramp*. I was very disturbed by comments like that, which meant to me that I would get worse. At least in their minds, they wanted to plan for the worst case scenario. I think pride kept me from ever wanting to be on display. Keep reading and you will see how humbled I have become. At that time, I began doing relaxation exercises every night after work. I would take ten deep breaths and say to myself, "I am in perfect, radiant health." I did this over and over again. I did not know Jesus at this time. I have learned that he is the answer, which I will share more fully later in this book.

Jeff and I were married in October 1991. My symptoms were gone, and I chose to forget about MS. I did not want to see anyone with the disease using a cane or in a wheelchair. I did not want to hear about or see anyone's symptoms because I feared I would get them too. Most people who knew me, including family, forgot I was ever diagnosed with MS.

My husband and I continued our regular travel. The hot islands did not bother me. I always had a determination in my heart that I was not meant to be sick. I wanted children, and I was working full-time. Therefore, I didn't have time to slow down. It is amazing to me now how my attitude has changed. I now have compassion for someone using assistance to perform life's normal activities. I now use things to help me, but at that time, I was not ready to even talk about MS or accept any help.

In September 1993, our son Dylan was born. What a blessing! Little did I know God would use him as the hands and feet for me when I needed them most. Dylan is a precious boy and very compassionate. I remember a time when I went to church on a Wednesday evening. Many times Dylan would stay with Jeff or my sister, and off I would go to church. On my way home, I was singing to praise and worship music in my car and hit a deer. I called my sister, who was watching Dylan, to tell her what had happened. Dylan was so concerned about me until I arrived home safely. I thank God Dylan has a very compassionate heart.

I questioned God why after I hit the deer. I now realize it is useless to ask God why and when. God will work it all out in his time, and whatever happens will be for our good. At fifty-five miles per hour, amazingly, my car was not badly damaged. I was unharmed and know the devil meant me harm. Thank God I was under his protection.

My life continued to be crazy. I worked full-time, and Dylan was in a family daycare. Jeff and I wanted more children. We tried, and I became pregnant in May 1995, only to miscarry six weeks later. I became pregnant three more times but sadly miscarried each one. By the time Dylan was four years old, I had lost four babies. The stress of it all started wearing on my health. Losing four babies was so devastating to us. Friends and relatives who had a child when Dylan was born went on to have their second child. It was hard to see what we wanted so badly and could not obtain. Jeff and I always wanted more children never wanting Dylan to be an only child. I felt as I had to give up the dream and desire for more children. I was emotionally undone. Dylan kept us going. God's grace is the only thing that got us through this time. We have come to appreciate the one gift he has given us: Dylan.

I started noticing numbness in my feet, but it did not stop me or slow me down. Little did I know God had other plans for me. Remember, sometimes God allows the fire (troubles and tribulation) to refine us. First Peter 1:6–7: "In this you greatly rejoice, though now for a little while you may have had to suffer grief in all kinds of trials. These have come so that your faith—of greater worth than gold, which perishes even though refined by fire—may be proved genuine and may result in praise, glory, and honor when Jesus Christ is revealed."

My World Changes as I Begin a New Journey

In August 1996, we decided to take Dylan on a vacation to the Cayman Islands. We made the long, hot trip with him, but when we got there, my husband was different. Jeff was a scuba diver, which was the main reason for visiting the islands. He didn't want to dive, tour the island, go to meals or swim in the ocean or pool with Dylan and me. His actions or lack of a desire to do anything was so different. We had traveled to the islands before, but I could not pinpoint what was wrong with Jeff. He was just not himself. After a few days, he came around. Jeff finally went diving while I stayed with Dylan on the shore. We swam either in the pool or in the ocean. I still wondered what was so different with my husband. We showed Dylan around the island, and things seemed to return to normal. We rented a scooter, and all three of us rode around touring the island. I still had numbness in my feet, but I refused to let it slow me down. Although we made it home in one piece, I was unprepared for the changes on the horizon.

Just one week later, I stopped at my parents to pick up Dylan, who was two years old at the time. He was running on their wet deck and fell. He refused to walk. Jeff came to my parents, and we decided to stop at the drugstore to get Children's Tylenol to ease his discomfort. We took him home and watched him crawl. I decided if there was no improvement in the morning, I would take him to the hospital.

In the middle of that night, my husband broke out in a deep sweat and experienced chest pain. He tossed and turned for hours. By 5:00 a.m., he told me to call my father to come and take him to the hospital. Fortunately, we were staying at our cottage that was minutes from my parents' home. I thank God for parents! My dad took Jeff to the hospital, and I planned to go to the hospital with Dylan as soon as he awoke.

My father called a couple hours later and informed me Jeff's EKG showed he had suffered a heart attack. I finally figured out why his behavior was so strange in the islands. I thank God Jeff did not have the heart attack while we were in the islands on vacation. Cayman Brac, where we stayed, has a very small hospital. Cayman Brac is one of the Cayman Islands that is only two miles wide and twelve miles long. The hospital would not have the ability to treat Jeff.

Dylan woke up, but he still would not walk, only crawl. Dylan never cried, only after he fell. I never imagined anything serious was wrong with his leg. I got Dylan together, picked up my mom, and headed to the local hospital. I arrived only to find out Jeff was being transported by ambulance to a larger hospital thirty minutes away. We decided to go on to the larger hospital and have Dylan checked out there with his dad. While driving to the larger hospital, I experienced a most awkward feeling. I had to pull over so the ambulance carrying my husband could pass. Never before did I feel so overwhelmed. Somehow during times like this, the adrenaline flowed, and I functioned. To look back and write about it now, it seems unbelievable. God was with me, but I didn't have a clue about God back then.

Upon arrival, I took Dylan to the emergency room, and the ambulance crew took my husband to the cardiac care unit. I was an emotional wreck! I thank the Lord my mother was with me. I ran back and forth between the emergency room and the cardiac care unit talking to doctors. Dylan's X-rays showed he had a break in his little, two-year-old leg. I bawled. How could I not know his leg was broken? He was put in a full cast, and my parents took him home with them.

I went back to the cardiac care unit (CCU) where Jeff was. I was unsure of what would become of Jeff. Jeff is a functioning alcoholic and I began to wonder if his alcohol drinking was the cause of his heart attack. When I met Jeff, he drank each night but that habit seemed "normal" to me as my parents have always had a drink each night before dinner. I really wanted to talk to his doctor to find out if his heart trouble was caused by his drinking.

Fortunately, he stabilized, and the doctor planned to do a heart catherization the following day with possible angioplasty. I was totally alone with no family or friends there with me. My parents would normally be there with me at the hospital. However, they were taking care of Dylan with his broken leg. I went to a phone booth, as cell phones were not yet popular, to call a friend that I worked with. I cried to her in such dismay and unbelief of what I was going through. I can recall feeling that my world was collapsing around me. Little did I know I would come to know a personal Savior named Jesus during this most stressful time.

My husband, Jeff, was in the hospital, and our son, Dylan, was recovering with my parents about thirty minutes away. I left the hospital exhausted and stopped to see a friend. She lived near our home and did reflexology (foot massage). I thought having my feet worked on might help my stress. During my appointment, my friend asked me if I had ever asked Jesus to come into my heart and take over my life. I wasn't sure what that meant, but I knew what I was going through was too much for me to handle. She told me all I had to do was pray, "Jesus, I know you died on the cross for my sins and rose from the dead. Come into my heart and take over. I cannot do this alone anymore." I actually prayed this prayer while driving my car shortly after leaving my friend's house on my way to pick up Dylan at my parent's house. You can ask Jesus into your heart anywhere at anytime. You might be saying, "What does this have to do with illness?" To conquer the battle of illness in your mind and totally change the way you look at your sickness, give your life to the Creator; it will bring you peace as you endure the storm. I have included the salvation prayer to ask Jesus in your life at the end of this book. In John 3:16, the Word says, "For God so loved the world that he gave his one and only son, that whoever believes in him shall not perish but have eternal life. For God did not send his son into the world to condemn the world but to save the world through him."

At that time in August 1996, I had no idea what was to come. All I knew was my life suddenly was turning upside down. I am thankful I did not have to go through this trial alone. Jesus is in control of my life since I accepted him as my personal savior. When I lived in the world before becoming a Christian, I was a sinner without a personal savior; but now because God sent his son to die on the cross for you and me, his blood covers my sins. God loves me unconditionally. I understand that after asking Jesus into my heart, when I do sin, I am forgiven as soon as I repent. Jesus died on the cross so that we can have everlasting life, so we may be healed, so we may prosper, and so we may be at peace. In John 14:27, the Word states, "Peace I leave with you, my peace I give to you. I do not give to you as the world gives." If you are reading this and have not asked Jesus to come into your heart and take over your life or maybe you do not have a clue what this all means, the first step toward healing physically, mentally, or emotionally can only begin with Jesus. He is the only way to heaven and the only way to fill the void in your life. His Word says in John 14:6, "I am the way and the truth and the life. No one comes to the Father except through me."

Jeff had angioplasty to open the artery in his heart that

caused his heart attack. I spoke to his doctor about his daily drinking affecting his heart but he did not see it as a problem. The doctor's response regarding his drinking was not what I wanted to hear. Five days later, Jeff was able to leave the hospital. I had real concern the nightly drinking would resume. At first he was a changed man, vowing he was not going to drink. He was happy to be alive, but the new revelation was short lived. At first he drank beer, but gradually liquor (gin) reappeared to his nightly routine. I was so hopeful that his drinking was a thing in the past. I have now realized what a sickness being addicted to alcohol can be and its affect on a family. As much as I tried, I could not change his problem.

After six weeks, Dylan got his cast off. Life seemed to return to normal, but soon it turned stressful all over again. Four months later, Jeff called me at work to tell me that he began having chest pain again and I needed to take him to the hospital. I took him to the same hospital. He had to undergo his second angioplasty. I could hardly believe he was having another procedure in only four months. Our business began to suffer, as he was out of work again. The stress of another medical procedure and not knowing how Jeff's heart would respond was unnerving. Dylan was three years old and thankfully did not understand his dad's condition.

It was April 1997, four months passed since Jeff's second angioplasty, and he began experiencing the same feeling once again in his chest. Somehow during each of these times I did not focus on the stress of it all. Each time, I called my place of work to take a personal day and drove him to the hospital. I was fortunate to work for an under-standing company.

Jeff refused treatment at the local hospital where they had performed two angioplasties in the prior eight months. He was transported by ambulance to another hospital thirty minutes away. I called my parents to pick up Dylan at daycare, and I drove to the hospital. Jeff had angioplasty for the third time. Jeff's angioplasty went well. His doctor told us that the other hospital where he had the two angioplasties likely got about fifty percent blood flow and sent him on his way. This is why the artery in his heart continued closing every four months. It has now been fourteen years, and thank God he has not had further heart trouble.

I found out during his last hospital stay that I was pregnant. I remember feeling very anxious wanting this baby to make it. I remember talking on a pay phone in the lobby of the hospital to my baby doctor, trying to be sure I was doing all I could to prevent another miscar-riage. I know the stress was too much for me to handle. Unfortunately, I went on to have my fourth miscarriage. This was difficult for Jeff and me because we always wanted two or three children. We decided to be thankful for the gift God gave us, namely Dylan. Not to say this was an easy time, however; we have learned to be thankful for what we do have. Dylan is a true blessing.

I think I was in a fog back then. To write about it all now seems so horrific. I made it through all of these trials only by the grace of God. I began to question why God was allowing us to go through such adversity. Considering all the stress, I had only minor MS difficulties at that time. I have come to realize God was with me and had an awesome plan even through this family fire. Do not let your circumstances make you fearful of the future. God says, "Do not fear for I am with you. Do not be dismayed for I am your God. I will strengthen you and help you. I will uphold you with my righteous right hand" (Isaiah 41:10). I continued working full-time, and because of my husband's health, our business was closed for weeks at a time. Therefore, we suffered financial difficulties.

I wondered if life would ever return to normal. I had a revelation while Jeff was hospitalized each time of how addicted to alcohol he was. Jeff would make a drink each night after work when he arrived home. I never thought this behavior was odd because my father always did the same thing. I started noticing during his hospital stays he was more and more eager to get home. He was hyper about getting released after the second and third angio-plasty. Upon arriving home, his first priority was to make a drink. I finally began to realize how serious his drinking had become and how addicted he was to alcohol.

I thank God for his grace that allowed me to endure this most stressful time. I now know God never left me.

My View of Illness Is About to Change

The MS that I believed was gone reappeared, and this time it would change my life completely . Jeff and I were having marital problems that were related to his addiction , so Dylan and I moved in with my parents. It was November 1999, and I was walking into work and fell. I was running late, carrying a gallon bottle of spring water, and tripped on the carpet inside the building. I fell face down, hitting the floor. I think the weight of the water pulled me forward, and I had no arms free to catch myself. My parents lived thirty minutes away, and I had taken Dylan to school. I was hurrying because it was 8:00 a.m., and I normally started work at 6:30 a.m. This was an extremely stressful time for all of us.

As a result of the fall, I was out of work for two weeks. During my recuperation time, I had an appointment at Family Court for a legal separation. My hope was that

Jeff would be forced to get help for his addiction. The Judge told Jeff he had to go to AA and a local alcohol rehab program. Jeff promised me he would seek help for his problem, and I believed him. Dylan and I moved back home. Once we were home, Jeff did not follow through on his word that he would get the necessary help. I have learned that he told me what I wanted to hear to get us home. I returned to work but started noticing my balance and gait were off a bit. I continued working until March 2000. I got to the point where it was hard to move. To walk around the office was a challenge. I ate lunch in my office and moved around very little. This was not easy because I had a very demanding job that required much movement. On March 20, 2000, I had a doctor's appointment with my internist. I told him I couldn't work unless he gave me something for my back because after the fall I had a lot of back pain. He checked my walk and told me my gait was off. He took me out of work, and I have not been back to work since. After two years on disability, I was terminated from my job, which was upsetting at the time, but I now know God had much better plans for me. I never thought I could be a stay-at-home mom. I had friends tell me I should stop working, and I would say, "I could never stay home because I would be so bored." Now, I wonder how I ever worked. Each day at home is full and rewarding. I think when you work full-time you just adapt to your schedule, and home stuff gets crammed into a few hours. I can honestly say I love being home and wonder how I ever felt different about working. Little did I know God had another plan for my life. Believe God's Word in

Jeremiah 29:11, which says, "For I know the plans I have for you declares the Lord, plans to prosper you and not to harm you, plans to give you a hope and a future."

I made myself an appointment with a local neurologist. It had been four years since my last neurological doctor's appointment. Remember that my previous neurologist was very positive. He told me when I would go see him with a concern that whatever problem I was having was not due to MS. He reminded me that I was diagnosed with a mild case of MS, and I would be fine. For years I forgot about MS, or at least I tried to forget about it.

Since my prior doctor had retired, it took me two weeks to get in to see the new neurologist. I had to repeat the MRI of my brain and other tests. When I met with Dr. Bhat, he confirmed that I had a lesion on my brain. It was located in the cerebellum, which affects balance. I knew that ten years ago I had no lesions (white spots) on my brain. My greatest fear was confirmed. I was prescribed daily injections of Copaxone. With no medical training, fear began to set in. The thought of giving myself a shot daily in different locations on my body scared me terribly. My world was turned upside down. I was weak and unable to do many things. But God had a plan far greater than I ever expected.

While I was home, I started studying God's Word. I began reading healing Scriptures. Suddenly, I began to have hope in what seemed hopeless. I realized healing was available to me. I continued appointments with my doctor. God made doctors, and we must use whatever means as God directs, such as medicine, therapy, items to help you, etc. Always remember our source for healing is God. The other items God may use, but ultimately he is the healer. When I began to understand that I did not have to be sick, I quoted the scripture in 1 Peter 2:24 which states "by his stripes I am healed." It is already done. However, one crucial thing to remember is healing belongs to us, but the manifestation is in God's timing. It has now been many years since I stopped working. Don't be discouraged if you don't get a miracle healing overnight. Once you are born again and ask Jesus to live in your heart, God will transform your life . You will realize you want his will more than anything. Your healing may take longer than you expect, but what you learn in the wait is well worth it.

I have learned that long-suffering produces endurance in your life. True long-suffering does not yield to anger, resentment, despair, or self-pity. In Romans 5:3, it says, "We also rejoice in our suffering because we know that suffering produces perseverance; perseverance, character, and character, hope. And hope does not disappoint us, because God has poured out his love into our hearts." Your attitude will determine your altitude. If you read Genesis 12, you will read God gave Abram (his name was later changed by God to Abraham, which means father of many nations) a promise that he would make him into a great nation, he would make his name great, and he would be a blessing. In chapter 15 of Genesis, God told Abraham a son would come from his body. He took him outside and told him to look up at the heavens and count the stars. "So numberless shall your offspring be." Abraham was seventy-five years old when God promised him a son. Their promise did not come to pass for twenty-five years. Can you imagine the thoughts Abraham and his wife Sarah must have thought? At their ages, they would conceive a child when Sarah was far beyond child-bearing age. God had a plan. Their old age did not stop God from bringing his promise to pass. Sometimes waiting on God can seem like forever; however, never give up hope.

Isaac was born when Abraham was one hundred years old. Can you imagine waiting twenty-five years for a promise? We all want magic and healing to drop out of heaven on us. I realized to wait upon the Lord in patience is the way to have peace in your storm. It will come to pass. God's timing is perfect. Abraham believed in hope at the promises God gave him. He did not waiver in unbelief regarding the promise, but he was strengthened as he gave praise and glory to God while waiting. As you give praise and glory to God despite your circumstances, you open the door for God's blessings. To receive the promise, you must endure the race with faith and patience and remain in the Word of God. God's promises regarding healing in his Word will come to pass in his timing. However, you must employ patient endurance during long-suffering that speaks and believes the Word of God despite adverse circumstances. I know I have struggled with the thief called time. I was so sure shortly after my disability began that God's Word was true, and it gave me such hope. I knew his promises were to me and every believer. However, as time has lingered, I have begun to doubt God. The devil wants us to believe his lies that God's promises will never come to pass. The devil is a liar. No matter how you feel, the doctor's report, or how long it takes to manifest, don't stop believing God's promises, no matter how long it takes. If God promised healing in his Word (which he did), it is not a matter of the promise; it is a matter of time. It surely will come to pass. It's only after you have prayed and developed a willingness to stand forever on the Word of God that you will receive what you asked of God and believed for in faith. I am doing the Lord's work and have come to realize that God has changed me through this sickness. I am now ready to help others with MS or other sicknesses. I am no longer afraid to hear of another person's symptoms because I know God has a good plan for my life. I will not live in fear. If you are in a place where it is hard to read this, remember perfect love casts out fear (1 John 4:18). God loves you and has made a way for you to be whole. As I stated earlier, I had such a fear of getting a symptom that someone else had that I did not want anything to do with MS or a person with MS. I hated to see someone struggle physically. I would avoid someone with a physical disability at all costs. There was one girl in the same building where I worked who had MS. She worked in a different location in the building, but from time to time I would run into her. I am always a positive encourager and was to her. However, seeing her struggle was difficult for me to see. Now, I find people look away from me and sometimes look in fear at me. Because of my relationship with God, I look at my situation so different. You or I cannot judge by what we see on the outside. What others may or may not think is unimportant. The reason my attitude has changed is because of Jesus. I am stronger on the inside than most. God created each of us for a special purpose. God's love has shown me he has an awesome plan for my life. You must put Jesus first in your life. Let him be the Lord of your life. His Word works for his children, those who have made him their Lord.

During my disability time, I have had many disappointments and at times have been very discouraged. I am currently working out once per week with a personal trainer. My lower body has become very weak, and I find standing to do normal activities like preparing dinner, washing dishes, putting on makeup, or blow drying my hair challenging. I always sit down. To God be the glory, I am getting stronger every day. I purchased a foldable scooter. What a blessing the scooter has been. My doctor told me in 2000 to purchase a scooter because it would save my energy and allow me to go places where I would have to walk long distances or stand for long periods of time. When you look at the devices such as a cane, wheelchair, walker, scooter, etc., as helpful tools while you wait upon God for his promises to come to pass, you can and will enjoy the ride, knowing God is greater than sickness.

It has taken me time, but I have learned that using items to assist you while you wait does not show a lack of faith. I never wanted special assistance, but what a blessing these items have turned out to be. You can be joyful right where you are, enjoying the journey on the way to where you are going. The flesh (world) will attempt to discourage you. Keep your eyes on God above. I have found it easier knowing God is in control. He has his eye on the clock and his hand on the thermostat, meaning he knows how much time we can take and how much heat we can endure. God won't let my trial (sickness) or yours last one moment longer than you or I can bear.

A friend told me a story that I always remember as I use assistance that God has provided. There was a man who was experiencing a terrible flood near his home. He prayed to God for help, yet over time he ended on his roof as the flood waters kept rising. Someone came to rescue the man by boat, but he refused to go. He told the rescuers, "I am believing God to send me help." He did not go in the rescue boat. Later, as the water continued to rise, another rescue boat came to take the man to safety. The man refused; again he chose to wait on God to save him. The man drowned and questioned God when he got to heaven asking why he did not save him. God told the man, "I sent two boats to rescue you, and you refused both".

The man was foolish, and he did not take the help God sent. Take help as needed. Stay positive and look at the help as a blessing. Victory will come, but don't be foolish, like this man was, while you wait.

What I Have Learned in the Fire

Finally, I realized that God was in control, and he would use all I've been through for his glory. This walk is hard, but "I can do everything through him who gives me strength" (Philippians 4:13). I have strength for all things in Christ who empowers me. I am ready for anything and equal to anything through him who infuses inner strength into me. I am self-sufficient in Christ's sufficiency.

Second Corinthians 12:9 says, "My grace is sufficient for you, for my power is made perfect in weakness." I depend upon the Lord. "In all your ways acknowledge him, and he will make your paths straight" (Proverbs 3:5–6).

Put first things first. There is healing available in Jesus. However, you cannot continue living a sinful life, praying once in a while and expecting God to move supernaturally in your life. When you are able, find yourself a church where you will be fed God's Word. Your spirit will be strengthened. Healing comes from the inside out. Every time I have blood work or a test, my results are perfect. You cannot go by feelings or what the outside looks like. Honestly, sometimes I await test results to get an answer to what the culprit is for why I feel as I do. To my surprise, my test results show everything is normal, and I realize healing does come from the inside out. My outer body has to line up with my inner body. All my test results show I am healed. By meditating and keeping the Word in your ears and before your eyes, healing will be the result. Romans 10:17 says, "Faith cometh by hearing and hearing by the Word of God." God wants you to prosper and be in health but it comes by strengthening and feeding your spirit the Word of the living God (KJV). Third John 2 states, "Dear friend I pray that you may enjoy good health and that all may go well with you even as your soul is getting along well." There was a time when I first became ill that I could not get to church. However, there are alternate ways to stay in the Word. I would watch Charles Stanley, Dr. Robert Schuller, Joel Osteen, or T.D. Jakes on Sunday mornings. Please understand I am not speaking of church in a religious sense. Your walk is not about religion, which, in many denominations, is made up of man-made rules and regulations. I am speaking of a personal relationship with Jesus Christ. The personal relationship is much more than out of guilt attending a church on Sunday mornings to meet an obligation, which is hopeless. Your walk will become a daily faith walk. I believe this is why many believe church is boring because they get nothing out of the service. How could a person ever live up to all the rules? Most religions teach and believe if you are a good person, you will go to heaven when you die. That belief is not in the Bible. I can speak of growing up Catholic and not truly knowing Jesus personally. I was bored silly in religion class. I went to church out of obligation but never experienced the personal relationship that I have now. I can say my walk with God is rewarding and is my choice not based on guilt or obligation. Your walk will be daily, not once per week. During the weekdays, I would and still watch Joyce Meyer, Kenneth Copeland, or Creflo Dollar. These shows are on early morning and excellent. I also listen to several audiotapes and, of course, spend much time reading the Bible. One tape that I listen to over and over again is Kenneth Hagin's tape titled, "God's Medicine." Most nights I go to sleep with the healing Scriptures playing on my CD player next to my bed. This is an excellent way to get God's Word on healing in you. I did and still wear a Walkman with the tape playing as I go through my day. If you are willing, there are many resources available to feed your spirit the Word of God.

In addition, when you are able, find yourself a church where you will learn and be fed God's Word. I now attend an Assembly of God church, which is such a blessing. I have grown tremendously since attending faithfully. I do have a dear friend who is unable to get to church because of health issues that prevent her from being around certain smells, such as perfume. However, she spends much of her time devoted to God's Word, trusting, and leaning on him. You can be committed to the Word and spend time with

God even if you don't get to church. God loves you even if you are unable to attend. Remember, the Bible is God's written word to us. I find reading the Bible to be my favorite time to spend, finding life in the Word of God. If you do not have a Bible, I suggest either a Living Bible, Amplified Bible, or NIV Bible. All the answers to your life's walk are in the book (Bible). It is like reading an awesome story, and all God's promises in the Bible are for the believer. During this fire, I have had much time on my hands, which allows me to grow up in my relationship with the Lord and know him personally. You will realize it is not about what the Lord can do for you but what he already did on the cross for you and me, which is more than enough. You just need to receive what he has already done. I have realized being healed was my primary focus, but my focus has changed. Along the way to healing, I realized knowing Jesus personally and praising him for all he has already done for me became my awesome privilege. When we stop striving and trying to get what he has already promised, you can just believe and leave the rest to God.

You see, I am on a shelf, so to speak. I am unable to perform life's daily activities. I can only look up. To say this time has been easy would be a lie. I often asked, "Why me? Why did you put me here?" God has a much bigger and better plan for us than we can even imagine. Only by the grace of God do I stay positive. I encourage others and instill hope in them. God is not the author of sickness; Satan is. If you are a believer, you are covered by an awesome God. He will only allow what is in your best interest to come upon you for your good and God's glory. He will see you through it. There may be sin in your life that caused your illness, but while God does not initiate it, he is in it if you are a believer. At times, he allows suffering to change us into what he created us to be. But remember a scripture I often remind myself of in Romans 8:28: "And we know that in all things God works for the good of those who love him, who are called according to his purpose." If you are not a believer, this does not include you, and you have reason for concern. Without God at the helm of your life, you have no covering, and Satan has full control over you and your health.

I am not mad at God for all I've been through and continue to go through. I realize questioning God is useless knowing he has a good plan for me. He will see me through. I am thankful he used this time to change me from the inside out. I would not change what I've been through. You may be thinking, *Oh, she must have had it much easier than me.* As you read on, I will share some of my struggle. As I go through this illness, I did not always know what I do now about God's Word. I am learning more all the time.

A few weeks after I stopped working, my son, Dylan, had the biggest event of the year at his school—a carnival. I was too weak to go, so he and my husband went. When they left, I cried and cried. You see, God blessed us with one child here and four in heaven. I hated to miss out on the fun time at his school carnival. While I was home in my recliner, I was reading healing scriptures. The Lord made one so alive to me! It was Isaiah 53:4–5, which says, "Surely he took up our infirmities and carried our sorrows, yet we considered him smitten by God, smitten by him and afflicted. But he was pierced for our transgressions, he was crushed for our iniquities, the punishment that brought us peace was upon him, and by his wounds we are healed."

I had read this scripture several times prior, but I suddenly realized he died for me so I may be healed. My time started out very sad that March night, but God turned it around to reveal his Word to me. My quiet times have been awesome because I have spent time getting to know God, developing a personal relationship with him.

This was just the beginning of my MS struggles, but God has never left me. His Word says in Hebrews 13:5, "Never will I leave you, never will I forsake you." I decided to go to an MS clinic and get another opinion. I was extremely nervous the day of the appointment. We had to travel two hours to a city to this MS clinic. The doctor was very thorough, and although I always keep a positive attitude, this clinic did much comparison with other MS patients. I found out at that time where the lesion was located on my brain that affected my balance and also affected my walking long distances and standing for long periods of time. Therefore, attending functions where I had to stand or walk any distance was a challenge. This caused me to miss out on Dylan's basketball games, festivals in the summer, carnivals, my husband's work parties and dinners, going to school for lunch with Dylan, etc. I couldn't walk into school to sign him out when I picked him up for an appointment. Dylan is now a teenager in high school, so that issue has come and gone. However, I really have come to realize I did not miss anything because God was working in me, growing me up spiritually. Don't think I didn't shed many tears knowing I could not do what most parents take for granted. I learned to trust in him and his timing. Each time, I got to know the Lord in awesome ways. This is not to say it was easy. I was very sad to miss out on activities with my husband and Dylan. Over time, I came to realize we are here for a short time, and eternity with the Lord will be far greater. I finally ordered a scooter and can go to functions at school or to the mall, etc. Our son is now in eleventh grade, and I remember many field trips I could not attend. It does not feel good to know I was home and available, but physically attending would be difficult. Also, there are times when Dylan goes to a function with a friend and their parents. I will ask him if he would prefer that I stay home versus him feeling uncomfortable with his mom being the only one on a scooter. I tell him it is okay to be honest if he would rather go with a friend. God always provides a way for him to go and gives me peace to endure staying home. Dylan is now a teenager, and I realize he does not want to be with his parents anyway; I know I was not hanging with my parents at his age. I am thankful for the precious times together and trust God to guide and watch over him when he is doing his things. Praise God I have been able to work on this book during his times away. The joy of the Lord is my strength (Nehemiah 8:10).

Grocery shopping, or any shopping, was a challenge, to say the least. It is very humbling to use one of those automatic shopping carts, but what a blessing from God. Dylan actually did not want me to use one, but once I did, he wanted to drive. He has liked to drive since he was a two-year-old on his Jeep ride-on toy. How we would laugh! Dylan would drive at times and run into stuff in the aisles. People looked at us as if we were crazy. Now God has blessed me with my own scooter. When Dylan goes shopping with me, he likes to drive and ride along. We make our times together fun times, knowing God ultimately is in control. Often, I have noticed people staring at me on my scooter trying to figure me out. I smile and many times encourage another to be thankful they have breath and a heart that is beating if they complain. Some people are most helpful, especially if I stand up and try to reach an item high on a shelf. However, there are those people who seem disgruntled and mad at the world. I believe all I have been through has humbled me. I now tend to appreciate every day and that my heart is beating. God wants us humble versus being full of pride, never stopping to appreciate the little things. If normal abilities are taken away from you, you will learn to be thankful in all things.

When I would go shopping prior to using a scooter to save my energy, I would come into the house and immediately lie down to rest. I would wait until Dylan or my husband got home so they could empty my car and carry the groceries in and put them away. I could only do one thing in one day and I was wiped out. Napping a couple times per day became a daily event for me. Still, today, I rest after lunch. I am up at 5:20 a.m. to do my devotion. Dylan is up for school by 6:00 a.m. and off to school by 6:45 a.m. I find I need a recharge after lunch. God knows when we sit, stand, lie down, arise, etc. The scripture that talks about this is found in Psalm 139. How awesome. God knows when we sit, stand, or even lie down. If you need to rest, God also gave us a brain, and we should refuel our bodies as needed. This does not mean you will always be required to nap daily.

I came to realize you cannot worry about what others think. That was hard for me. I was always insecure and never wanted to be in the spotlight. I realized God doesn't always change the circumstances. He wants to change us first. At times when I could go to some events, walking into my son's school for a parade or basketball game was a challenge because all the moms and dads remembered me running one hundred miles per hour. They were walking by sight and not by faith!

I learned that my cane was my rod and my staff. Psalm 23 says, "Your rod and your staff they comfort me." So I saw it as my sword. After a woman's conference at our church, a group of ladies went to Friendly's for ice cream. It was late, and we were all in a silly mood. I had to go to the bathroom, and I got hysterical laughing. Have you ever noticed when people see a cane or wheelchair, they back up and act like a huge semi or tractor-trailer coming through, and they get out of the way. People do it no matter where I am. Well, that night at Friendly's, my girlfriend and I went to the bathroom, and I held up my cane as people got out of the way like always and said, "On guard, this is my sword." We could laugh and enjoy the moment because when you know your God and what his Word says, the response of others really does not matter. I do not want to minimize the fact that at times others can hurt you by looks or remarks. I now realize how precious other people are, and all I have been through has made me very humble in my dealings. I now look at others with disabilities with a compassion I did not have before my own struggle. Before, I was like many of the people in the world who are always in a hurry, never thinking of others before myself. I realize how unfortunate and sad I was and many people are. They appear all together on the outside, but without Jesus, life ultimately is very empty and shallow. You will feel sorry for the lost souls and appreciate your relationship with God, which is far greater than anything this world has to offer. It should not matter what others think, for God says, "You dear children are from God and have overcome them because the one who is in you is greater than who is in the world" (1 John 4:4). Jesus in us is much greater than Satan, who is the author of sin and sickness in this world. With Jesus in you, it does not matter what the world thinks. If you are trusting Jesus as the Lord of your life, keep smiling!

I realize as a believer all things that happen are "father filtered," meaning nothing comes near you that God doesn't allow for your good. Genesis 50:20 says, "But God intended for good." All that I have gone through is God's perfect plan for my life. I did not always believe as I do now. It has been a process to come to know and pray for his will for me over all else. I have taken much time to believe God's Word and let my faith trust that Jesus already paid the price and it is done. Many of us ask God to do whatever we pray about, but we do not believe he heard us or that it is done. We try to help him, get others to help, and anxiously wait to see how he is going to work. I now pray, believe he is working, and take my hands off, leaving God time to work. This is not always easy to do but trusting God knows best is the only way.

I know many of you reading this that may have been diagnosed with MS may have a hard time inching along to avoid reading anything on MS. You may have a fear of this happening to you. I have been in your shoes. Before this fire (sickness), I was in denial of MS. I had a fear of ending up like someone else who seemed worse off than me. Now, I notice others with MS or some disability that cannot look at me on my scooter . When you have a personal relationship with Jesus, you can look at others with confidence. I feel sad for them if they do not know Jesus as their personal Savior and the healer as I do. I have learned to cheer up! Jesus came so that we might have and enjoy life and have it more abundantly. Keep your focus on Jesus and what he promises in his Word. I mentioned we had a cottage. For four summers, I felt like I lived in a fish bowl. Our cottages are very close to one another. Every neighbor seemed to know of my illness without ever seeing me or my struggle. My husband had a hard time dealing with the changes in my life and told many of the neighbors at the lake what I was dealing with. Being a private person, suddenly I parked my car down the hill (an obvious change) next to the cottage because it was a distance to walk down our steps or down the hill to the door. The laundry at the lake was in the basement, and we had two neighbors next door who would stare at me as I tossed the laundry basket down (so I didn't put additional strain on my back). I learned to put my spiritual blinders on and go about my chores. The neighbors offered to help, but I was determined to do it myself. They did not understand my faith or my determination, and I did not want to submit to needed help. I have learned it is humbling but a blessing to be offered help. I began to accept the help. Don't be too proud, as I was, to ask and receive needed help.

We also had many steps to go down to the water. Our handrail needed to be replaced, and I could not walk down without holding on. I begged my husband to replace it, but he said we did not have the money. We had an elevator that went down the bank to the lake, and Jeff wanted me to use it. I wanted to be independent and get what little exercise I could. My husband felt I did not want to be seen on the elevator by the neighbors. Needless to say, I used the elevator for two years. It was hard because the elevator was very loud, and I felt everyone knew my coming and going. Also, I truly wanted the exercise. I knew I could walk down if the handrail was replaced even if it took me much longer than in the past.

If you are married, you may or may not have a supportive spouse. I have to say that dealing with my husband's negativism toward my illness was stressful and hard. He could not understand my faith because he was not walking the same faith walk with me. Through my disability, Jeff had not been the most supportive. He would constantly tell me, "You are in denial. You are not getting better. You will be in a wheelchair." Each time I had to listen to him, I would say, "God is greater than MS. You will not take my hope from me; by his stripes I am healed" (1 Peter 2:24). It was a challenge and still is, for we are unequally yoked. I'm living in the kingdom, walking by faith, but he is living in the world, walking by sight. I pray continually for Jeff's salvation. I know God's Word says, "But as for me and my household, we will serve the Lord" (Joshua 24:15). I often wonder what it would be like to have a supportive spouse regardless of my physical condition. In Scripture, the Word states that God will be your husband. When your husband is not being the husband God created him to be, God is faithful and will be a husband to you and take great care of you and meet all your needs. In Isaiah 54:5, the Word states , "For your maker is your husband—the Lord Almighty is his name."

If you are in a similar place as I have been, where your spouse speaks negative words to you, remember God loves you. Jeremiah 31:13: "I have loved you with an everlasting love." Romans 5:5, "And hope does not disappoint us because God has poured out his love into our hearts." Never give up hope. You do not have to receive garbage into your spirit. Just keep your eyes on Jesus. I know this trying time is also difficult on Jeff. I have not been able to do all the things I used to, but he is blinded by the god of this world. I know that a praying wife is very powerful. I often tell Jeff that he has a praying wife when he will tell me of something good that has happened to him

Do not lose heart if you don't have the most supportive and understanding spouse. God is faithful, and I continue to stand on his Word and promises. If your family, friends, or spouse do not understand your faith and strength, remember "the one who is in you is greater then the one in the world" (1 John 4:4). I have included healing scriptures in the last chapter of this book. Study them, speak them aloud to yourself, and claim them. First Peter 2:24 says, "He himself bore our sins in his body on the tree so that we might die to sins and live for righteousness; by his wounds you have been healed." The stripes were the thirty-nine lashes Jesus took before he was crucified. I have to say Jeff has realized he cannot shake my faith, and although he doesn't understand it, he no longer speaks negatively about my future. Keep praying for your unsaved loved ones. I stand on the scripture in Joshua 24:15, which says, "But as for me and my household, we shall serve the Lord." God will hear and answer your prayers.

MS can be difficult when you see it, or any illness, through the world's point of view. Keeping a positive attitude and trusting God each day has helped me tremendously. In addition, I know nutritional supplements have helped me replace nutrients that my body needs to function. Take steps to make your life a bit easier during your illness time. Recently, we've hired someone to clean. This is a tremendous help and allows me to spend time in God's Word and time to write. Since we sold our cottage, where it was normally cooler in the summer, I purchased two window air conditioning units. What a blessing on those hot and humid days.

I have experienced many different emotions dealing with family. My parents, brother, and sister are very supportive. Not only did they help me financially, they are also there for me emotionally and physically. I know this is difficult for the7m; however, they do not understand my faith. I believe they think my church is getting me through this time, but my personal relationship with Jesus is the reason I do not give up. It is not about a church. I am walking by faith, not by sight. Jesus is why I press on through adversity. I know my family is concerned about my well-being. I truly am trusting the one who knows all our days and, I believe, will work it all out for good.

I started going to a naturopath doctor who helped me find nutritional deficiencies in my body. You see, MS means multiple deficiencies. I will address this in more detail in a later chapter. These appointments were costly for me and not covered by insurance. My parents blessed me, and I was able to pay the cost. My parents and siblings also paid for a contractor to build a new handrail and steps at our cottage. My husband bought the materials, and my family paid the contractor. In the middle of the summer 2001, I felt free. I was able to walk down to the lake at my pace, thanks to my family's generosity. My extended family (aunts, uncles, and cousins) were supportive also. In October 2000, I was running late taking my son to my cousin's house for a birthday party. When I got to the house, I noticed the driveway was open so I could pull up and let Dylan out without having to get out of the car. When I pulled in, my foot felt glued to the gas pedal, and we drove right through the garage. There were parents and kids all around. I thanked God that no one was hurt. My son and I were okay, just shook up. My cousin and his wife were very loving and understanding. My cousin did call the police for insurance reasons. A friend of mine had stopped to visit before we left for the party. Dylan and I were late, and we needed to be on time, as the kids were going to a pool to swim. I was speeding rushing to get there.

While I sat in the driveway waiting for the police to arrive, all the parents had gone into the house. I waited and cried. I am sure they all blamed MS for the accident. I was very humiliated and had to listen to criticism suggesting that I needed controls on my steering wheel or maybe I shouldn't drive. I prayed to God and asked him to reveal to me if I shouldn't drive, especially when Dylan was with me. . The Lord spoke to me, "You will be fine, just slow down." Once you are saved, God will speak to you. You must get quiet and listen. When times like this happen, God is still on the throne and in control. Try to look at the positive in every situation. He protected me from harming another child or adult. As time went on, the talk ceased, and I resumed driving. However, for months I was nervous while driving. I gave up my hurriedness and slowed down, enjoying the journey. If you happen to be late to an event, don't push yourself and cause an unnecessary accident. Remember to pray always. If you are late, God can make it all work for your good.

It is awesome to have a personal relationship with Jesus. You may wonder why I included this story. I want you to know some of what I have been through, and it was not always easy or comfortable. I even had a cousin say to my mom after this accident, "Her brain is not telling her foot what to do." My mom was in tears. My parents are Catholic and do not understand all the promises in God's Word, such as healing. My parents pray and go to church, and I know that seeing me deal with this sickness has been difficult for them. However, I have stood on God's Word, and I am walking by faith, not by sight. Second Corinthians 5:7 says, "For we walk by faith not by sight" (KJV). Many others walk by sight, and even now as I use my scooter, many do not know how to take my positive attitude. I recently went to physical therapy at a local hospital. Physical therapy is on the eighth floor, and I used my scooter to get there. The distance is so far that I would be exhausted walking. When I was on my way to my appointment in the elevator, I would always speak my faith and positive encouragement to others. My scooter is foldable and rather small. It draws much attention, and people always ask about it, which gives me an opening to speak about the Lord. I feel privileged to have the opportunity to show the joy of the Lord to a dying world. God has a good plan. I know in my heart God knows best. "For I know the plans I have for you, declares the Lord, plans to prosper you and not to harm you, plans to give you hope and a future" (Jeremiah 29:11).

One thing I know for sure: healing is a promise in God's Word. The manifestation of your healing takes place in God's time, not yours or mine. I have had hands laid on me, been in healing prayer lines, stood on God's Word, etc. Speaking the Word out of your mouth is the most vital part of receiving your healing. Find promises in God's Word and make them personal (put your name in the scripture). For example, he took Karen's infirmities and bore Karen's sicknesses. You must believe the Word and expect his promises to manifest in your body. Healing belongs to the believer, but sometimes God uses these times to refine us to be used for his kingdom. God will either perform a miracle, heal in his time, or take us home to heaven. He knows best. Don't give up speaking and believing his promises; keep on keeping on until the physical manifestation appears. I have been changed, and if God had healed me instantly, I would not have slowed down to get to know the Lord by spending time in his Word, write this book, smell the roses, and appreciate every day that I get out of bed. Remember, it is not a matter of the promise in God's Word; it is a matter of the time. His timing is perfect. Isaiah 40:31 states, "They that wait upon the Lord shall renew their strength, they shall mount up with wings as eagles; they shall run and not grow weary; they shall walk and not faint" (KJV). I have had several disappointments, continually having to stay positive. People often pity me and my circumstance. I try to speak positive words to them, but honestly I do get tired of always feeling like I have to defend my faith.

When you begin to feel discouraged and doubt God , trust him with all your heart, and his promises will come to pass. Don't lose your hope. "Hope deferred makes the heart sick" (Proverbs 13:12). Don't focus on the symptoms or how you feel. Keep your focus on God's Word and off yourself. "Delight yourself also in the Lord and he will give you the desires and secret petitions of your heart" (Psalm 37:4, AMP). Don't go by feelings. Go only by God's Word. It is not about how you feel, but it is about whom you know (Jesus). Speak the healing promises out of your mouth, and you will see healing come to pass.

Remember, we get what we speak, either good or bad. Always speak the positive. "Reckless words pierce like a sword but the tongue of the wise brings healing" (Proverbs 12:18).

Nutrition 101

For many years, I have taken nutritional supplements, but when I became ill, I realized how vitally important it is to give your body proper nutrition. Multiple sclerosis and many illnesses really mean multiple deficiencies. We need more nutrition than healthy individuals. It is very difficult to get all your nutrition from your food, especially when you consider the typical American diet. Proper supplementation is necessary, and the type of vitamins needed varies from individual to individual.

I will explain what I have done to maintain my health, and I firmly believe I will see victory over illness, first due to the Lord and secondly, due to proper nutrition. Feed your body properly, and God will take care of the rest. There are many choices in vitamins, but they are not all good quality. I use Shaklee, Life Extension, Thorne Research, and Standard Process. Be careful which brand you choose. Although some brands are less expensive, they may not be whole food supplements, not of good quality, or not easily digestible.

Below, I have listed the supplements I take. I will explain in detail those that I believe are most essential for our bodies.

Multivitamin with iron	CoQ10
Protein	Free Forming Amino Acids
B complex	Lecithin
Digestive Enzymes	Vitamin C
Probiotic	EPA/DHA
Vitamin E	Calcium and Magnesium

In someone with MS, myelin sheath deficiency can be found in the brain or spinal cord (white spots on an MRI show lesions where myelin is missing). Myelin sheath is made up of essential fatty acids, protein, and lecithin. I believe the following supplements are essential to help rebuild the myelin sheath that is covering the nerves.

Protein

Protein is an important component of every cell in the body. This is an essential part of nutrition, second only to water in the body's physical composition. Proteins make up 20 percent of our body weight and are a primary component of our muscles, hair, nails, skin, eyes, and internal organs, especially the heart muscle. Our immune system defense requires protein for the formation of antibodies that help fight infection.

Essential amino acids are those our body cannot synthesize on its own and which we must acquire through our diet. I take Shaklee Soy Protein, which contains nine essential amino acids per serving.

I began taking Copaxon (a daily shot for MS) in March 2000. The reason I agreed to take it was because it was the only noninterferon drug for MS. The make-up of Copaxon is four synthetic amino acids that, to me, sounded better than the interferon drugs that had adverse side effects. I know people with MS who take shots of interferon drugs. Many of them are so much worse off. Many stay in bed much of the time because the shots cause flulike symptoms. I do not want my immune system suppressed with an interferon drug. I have not spent a day in bed for nine years. To think of a drug causing symptoms that may make me worse is a chance I am not willing to take. I believe feeding your body proper nutrition, adequate rest, and a positive attitude is crucial to winning the battle.

The T cells in someone with MS attack the mylein sheath, causing lesions. Copaxon is believed to act as a buffer so the T cells attack the Copaxon instead of the myelin sheath. Since I started taking a protein drink supplement each day that contains nine natural essential amino acids, I no longer take my daily shot of Copaxon. Since I am feeding my body amino acids daily, I found I no longer needed synthetic amino acids. In addition to the protein drink, I use free-forming amino acids in capsule form in the morning on an empty stomach. The amino acids are called Metaplex by Thorne Research. Originally, I obtained them from my doctor's office. Since then, I order them from a vitamin distributor. A local pharmacy also carries Metaplex. Metaplex contains the four natural amino acids that Copaxon includes synthetically. If anyone puts something in his body that is not needed, it turns toxic in your system. I stopped my shots in October 2001. I would not suggest you stop taking medicine just because I did. It's important to trust God's timing before stopping any medication when you feel it is time. As you grow in your relationship with the Lord, he will direct your steps. Lean on, trust in, and be confident in the Lord with all your heart and mind, and do not rely on your own insight or understanding (Proverbs 3:5, AMP).

Every part of our bodies relies on protein for proper growth and normal functioning. Supplementing with protein is vital, as it is the stuff we are made of.

Lecithin

Lecithin is an oil found in most living tissues. It is important for many body functions, particularly healthy nerves and cell membranes. Nerve and brain cells depend on their nourishment chiefly from lecithin. Lecithin has been found to be an essential part of the brain, nervous system, endocrine glands, and the muscles of the heart. Lecithin deficiency is a common problem in many, and adding lecithin to your diet can help starved nerves and glands return to normal functioning. Lecithin helps your body metabolize fats and acts as a fat emulsifier. People with MS can have a deficiency of lecithin in the brain and the myelin sheath that covers the nerves. I believe lecithin is a vital supplement for optimal health in the brain and nervous system.

EPA/DHA

To protect the myelin sheath against a deficiency of essential fatty acids, I take EPA with DHA (fish oil capsules). This oil helps to suppress autoimmune reactions and provides the building blocks to help rebuild the myelin sheath. Essential fatty acid EPA (omega-3) can be a helpful addition to your supplement program, but always check with your doctor or a nutritionist to see what is right for you.

Vitamin D

This vitamin is vital for the proper development of the nervous system and poorly constructed neural tissues that may break down in later years. Calcium is dependent on vitamin D for its utilization. Vitamin D can be obtained from exposure to sunlight. Living in the northern states, we do not always have adequate amounts of sunshine. Vitamin D has numerous effects on the immune system and acts with the central nervous system. A person needs to supplement calcium and magnesium with vitamin D supplementation.

CoQ10

This supplement is used to provide energy in the cells. It transfers electrons in the cells in the mitochondria that produce energy to help the cells. I take fifty milligrams a day.

I take additional vitamins as seen on my list at the

beginning of this chapter. I believe they are all beneficial to overall health. I explained in detail those I believe
are most beneficial to someone dealing with illness or
disease. Every one of us is different, so be sure to check
with a nutritionist or your health care professional prior
to beginning any supplementation. Over the years, I have
changed my vitamin regime many times. I now realize
how vital being consistent with your supplements is to
one's health. I have gone through my share of struggles,
but I now realize I could be much worse off if I were not
faithful to feed my body properly. Be consistent with your
supplements each day; consistency is important to rebuild
you health. It takes discipline but will pay off in the end.

What You Eat and Drink Does Make a Difference

Water, Water, Water

Approximately two-thirds of a person's body weight is water. Our blood is 82 percent water. Both our brain and muscles are 75 percent water. I cannot stress enough the importance drinking water (preferably spring or filtered). Water is the primary component of all our bodily fluids, including blood, lymph, digestive juices, urine, tears, and sweat. Water is involved in almost every bodily function: circulation (a must in MS), digestion, absorption, and elimination of wastes. Water is fundamental to all life on Earth. Without clean water, we cannot experience optimal health. Be careful in choosing your drinking water. I drink spring water and rarely drink tap water. You really don't know where that water comes from or what it may be contaminated with. You need at least one half your body's weight in ounces of water per day. For example, if you weigh one hundred pounds, you should drink fifty ounces of water per day. If you do not like water alone, try a slice of lemon or lime in it. I gave up coffee and soda years ago. Water is the main thing I drink. Once in a while, I drink a cup of green tea that you can buy with or without caffeine.

If you don't drink enough water, you could become dehydrated especially on those hot summer days. You can also slow down your metabolism and may experience day-time fatigue. Are you drinking enough water?

Soda Pop

You may drink soda pop and consider that your daily intake of liquid, however, soda pop is full of sugar and horrible for your system. Soda pop is liquid candy for any-one who drinks it—adults and children alike. Soda pop is Americans' single biggest source of refined sugars. Soft drinks provide the average male with 15 teaspoons of sugar a day and the average female with about 10 teaspoons a day. Obviously these amounts will increase if someone drinks higher amounts of soda per day. One of every four drinks consumed is a soft drink. Sugar, such as that in soda pop, has a greater effect than other carbohydrates on raising triglyceride levels in the blood. Sugar can suppress the immune system and upset the body's mineral balance.

With any illness, people have weakened immune systems without adding sugar. Sugar further weakens the immune system. When you choose to drink soft drinks, you are compromising your own immune system ever further. Sugar can also weaken your defense against bacterial infections. Sugar can also exacerbate the symptoms of illness. We need to keep our pH around 7.0. Sugar is an acidic food and will make it more difficult to maintain the proper pH. We need to eat and drink more alkaline foods and drinks. I will explain further in this chapter.

When you realize how soda pop may be adversely affecting your health, it is easy to change from choosing soda to water, which is a much healthier choice. Each daily soda pop also increases your obesity risk by 60%. Remember MS means multiple deficiencies. Soda is one of the main nutritional reasons most people suffer from health problems. It parallels alcohol in one profound similarity. If one drinks all that sugar in soda pop, the appetite is relatively suppressed from nourishing foods like fruits and vegetables, which results in nutritional deficiencies. Think twice before you pop open your next can of soda pop.

Diet Products

You may be thinking, "I'm okay. I drink diet soda." However, most diet soda contains aspartame. Aspartame is not a diet product. It will make you crave carbohydrates and can make you fat. This is marketed as Nutrasweet, Equal, Spoonful, etc. Aspartame can cause many health problems including methanol toxicity that mimics multiple sclerosis. There are 92 documented symptoms of aspartame. It would be wise to Google aspartame and its effects on health and research for yourself to see if you want to consume this product. There are other options such as stevia and xylitol that can be used as a sweetener vs. sugar or a product containing aspartame.

Eating Healthy

Through my sickness and for a time before, I have become very cautious about what I eat. My doctor recommended the Swank Diet be incorporated into my eating habits. This diet is very strict concerning the dietary intake of fats. It is referred to as a low-fat diet with a 90 percent reduction of fat intake as compared to the typical American diet.

Fruits and vegetables are vitally important too. I recently had a blood test through my doctor (internist). The blood test is called Elisa Act. The test checks the blood for any food allergies and anything that may weaken your immune system. I found out that my body was too acidic and I needed to eat more alkaline foods. Our pH should be about 7.0. Therefore, I needed to change my eating and drinking. Acidic foods are much easier to grab when we are on the go. The lab sent me the book *The Alkaline Way*, which teaches you how and what to eat to make your body's pH balanced. If your body is too acidic, it is difficult to be healthy. We definitely need a balance of acidic and alkaline foods. I will list a few items that are alkaline foods you can add to your diet:

pineapple	limes	lemons
pumpkin seeds	sweet potatoes	yams
tangerine	raspberry	watermelon
garlic	asparagus	broccoli
grapefruit	cantaloupe	potato
cauliflower	cabbage	eggplant
almonds	cashews	

You need to eat a variety of foods. A balance of foods is the best way to live a healthy life. When we are busy and on the go, it is easy to grab prepared foods instead of healthy fruits and vegetables. It all takes discipline, but it is well worth it to walk in divine health.

High-fat foods should be eliminated and replaced with foods containing unsaturated fatty acids. I try to avoid trans fats, processed sugars, alcohol, and white flour. Many companies have recently eliminated trans fat in their food items. Beware of fast food restaurants. The French fries are normally cooked with trans fat. I pray all restaurants will eliminate this artery-clogging oil. I rarely eat beef and never eat pork. I do eat chicken (minus the skin) and fish, which is excellent for someone with MS. I bake or broil, and I rarely eat fried food.

In place of milk, I drink soy milk. Soy contains phytonutrients called isoflavones that are wonderful for one's overall health. When shopping, be careful when buying foods such as packaged lunch meat, cake mixes, muffins, cookies, brownies, cheeses, pastries, and other processed items. They contain hidden or unknown quantities of transsaturated fat. Eating fresh fruits and vegetables (especially raw) along with whole grain breads and cereals is beneficial for everyone. A low-fat diet is beneficial for all of us, not just someone dealing with a chronic illness. If you want to be well, watch what goes into your mouth. It is worth it!

Parasites

In July 2001, I went to my six-month neurologist appointment. I had a very positive appointment with my doctor. Both my upper body and lower body were stronger. The one thing that concerned my doctor was I had lost weight since my last checkup. I was looking anorexic and didn't even realize how I looked. I normally weighed 110 pounds, but at that time, I was just ninety-two pounds. My doctor wanted to see me again in six months and told me I had to gain five pounds. My appointment was on a Tuesday, and I prayed afterward for God to reveal why I was losing weight. The next night, I went to Wednesday night service at church, and we had an altar call for anyone who needed renewed hope. I, of course, went up to the altar and, unknown to me, while I was at the altar, two women in the congregation were praying for me. They saw me looking so sick and thin, using my cane to get around. After the altar call, a friend of mine spoke to these women. They both had a word for me from the Lord. I went to see them immediately after the service. They told me that the Lord showed them that I was covered with parasites (in my body). The parasites were eating all my nutrients and leaving me the junk. They gave me the name of a doctor that could verify if I, in fact, had parasites. Shortly after, I got in to see the doctor, and it was confirmed. I became extremely thin and weak. My muscles were depleting. It has taken me a lot of time to rebuild my muscles with the help of friend who is personal trainer. Finally, my muscles were returning. God is so good. I prayed the day before for an answer to my weight loss, and the next night, I had an answer to that prayer. One day, I saw pictures of myself during the time I had parasites, and I could not believe how I looked.

Getting checked out by a naturopath doctor is well worth it. Many doctors do not check or know how to check for parasites. A parasite lives a parallel life inside our bodies, feeding off our own energy, our cells, or the food we eat and/or the health supplements we use. Unfortunately, medical testing procedures only catch about 20 percent of the cases of parasites. I had no idea I was losing weight and muscle due to parasites. Many people get alarmed when they hear *parasites*. They think of a dog with worms, but when your immune system is compromised and your body is under stress, parasites can become a silent health problem. After I completed a three-month parasite cleanse, I was free of parasites. If you suspect you may have parasites, it is well worth it to be checked. If you find out you do have them, here are some foods to add to your diet and others to avoid. I learned to control stress in my life and watch everything I ate during this time.

Foods to Add:

- Pumpkin seeds
- Garlic
- Apple cider vinegar
- Cranberry juice

Foods to Avoid

- Raw or uncooked fish, beef, pork, or chicken
- Cooked pork, bacon, ham
- Sugar and carbohydrates
- Water chestnuts
- Unwashed fruits or vegetables, or those washed in questionable water

Candida Albicans

Another area I have had to deal with is *Candida albicans* (yeast overgrowth). Everyone has Candida, a form of yeast normally confined to the lower bowels, the vagina, and the skin. In healthy individuals with strong, functioning immune systems, it is harmless and kept in check by good bacteria called bifidobacteria and acidophilus. However, if your immune system is compromised (as in disease or illness), the Candida yeast can turn into an aggressive fungus that can infect other body tissues and compromise one's health. This is called candidiasis.

As I walked through this MS fire, I came to realize yeast overgrowth was affecting my health. There are many symptoms associated with Candida, and some mimic MS. I dealt with chronic fatigue, drowsiness, bloating, constipation, heartburn, sensitivity to odors, perfumes, smoke, etc.

My naturopath doctor confirmed I was fighting Candida. In order to overcome candidiasis, I had to avoid sugar in all forms. I used an acidophilus supplement to balance my intestinal environment with beneficial good bacteria. I took Candex by Pure Essence Labs, which is made up of enzymes to control Candida.

Candidiasis can add to the stress on individuals with illness. It is worth it to find out from your doctor if *Candida albicans* may be affecting your overall health and adding to your health difficulties. Candida can be detected by a stool sample.

It's Well Worth It

As you have read, I have dealt with many things that compromised my health. Consequently, I have become very disciplined in my eating and drinking because I find it necessary to combat disease and strive for wellness. It is not always easy, but it is most beneficial to say, "No, thank you" to the birthday cake, a glazed donut, or sweets. When you see others eating and drinking whatever they want and you have to be so disciplined, it can be hard at the time; however, it will pay off in good overall health. What a blessing last Thanksgiving when my sister-in-law made a pumpkin pie with stevia as a sweetener in the place of sugar. You really cannot taste the difference. Remember, many people will eventually have some health problem down the road if they continually abuse their bodies with sugar, fatty foods, soda, alcohol, smoking, and on and on. You may feel like the only one who declines certain foods or drinks, but the outcome and payoff will be well worth it. Pray that God will take away the temptations from you and that your body will become a vessel used for his glory. Also, remember if you have made Jesus the Lord of your life by asking him to come into your heart and take over, the Holy Spirit lives on the inside of you. Your body is the temple, which needs to be taken care of appropriately. You will be rewarded for your obedience, even in eating and drinking. I can say now, as many years have passed, I do occasionally treat myself to a sweet but use wisdom, knowing how stress and particularly sugar adversely affected my health in the past.

"Do you not know that your body is the temple of the Holy Spirit who is within you, whom you have received from God? You are not your own. You were bought with a price. Therefore, honor God with your body" (1 Corinthians 6:19–20).

The Key

By now I hope you have come to realize what the key is to overcoming MS or any other illness. The key is Jesus Christ. He came to the earth to destroy the works of the devil. "The thief (Satan) comes only in order to kill and destroy. I (Jesus) came that they may have and enjoy life and have it in abundance" (John 10:10, AMP).

God is not the author of sickness. Satan is. Asking Jesus into your heart to be the Lord of your life is the only way to have victory. You do not have to settle for sickness, be it MS, cancer, lupus, or any other disease. Sometimes God allows us to go through the fire (sickness), but he will never leave us nor forsake us. "Neither will I leave you; never will I forsake you" (Hebrews 13:5). He did not initiate the sickness; however, he is with you if you have dedicated your life to him. He will see you through the sickness and beyond.

For me, this illness changed me totally. I came to realize God is in control and will work all things together for good for those who love him (read Romans 8:28). Waiting on God has been challenging, but I know patience is being worked out in me. I am sharing in Christ's suffering. "Now if we are his children then we are heirs—heirs of God and co-heirs with Christ, if indeed we share in his sufferings in order that we may share in his glory" (Romans 8:17). When you look at your sickness from God's perspective, he ultimately knows best. The wait is bearable. Stand on the Word found in Isaiah 40:31: "He gives strength to the weary and increases the power of the weak. Even youths grow tired and weary and young men stumble and fall but those who hope in the Lord will renew their strength. They will soar on wings like eagles; they will run and not grow weary, they will walk and not faint."

When I realized God was in control of my life, I no longer had the fear of MS getting worse. I know God will see me through every obstacle and challenge. When you finally understand the awesome healing power available to every believer, you can rest in the Lord. "When you pass through the waters, I will be with you, and through the rivers they will not overwhelm you. When you walk through the fire, you will not be burned or scorched, nor will the flame kindle upon you" (Isaiah 43:2, AMP). God's Word is awesome. All God's promises in his Word (the Bible) are for you and me as believers. In the book of Daniel chapter three, King Nebuchadnezzar ordered Shadrach, Meshach, and Abednego to worship him. Because they did not, he cast them into a fiery furnace. They would not worship anyone except God. They believed their God was able to deliver them from the fiery furnace. Nebuchadnezzar was full of fury and commanded these three men to be bound and cast into the fiery furnace. He commanded that the furnace be turned up seven times hotter than it usually was. Shadrach, Meshach, and Abednego fell down bound into the burning furnace. Because the furnace was exceedingly hot, the flames and sparks killed the men who put Shadrach, Meshach, and Abednego into the furnace. King Nebuchadnezzar was astounded when he saw four men loose, walking in the midst of the fire. They were not hurt. They came out, and the fire had no power upon their bodies, nor was the hair on their heads singed. They did not even smell like smoke. The fourth man in the furnace with them was Jesus.

Just as the story reveals, God was with Shadrach, Meshach, and Abednego in the fire. They came out unharmed. God will be with you during your fiery trial. How awesome they did not even smell like smoke. "Jesus Christ is the same yesterday and today and forever" (Hebrews 13:8). These men worshipped God in the midst of controversy, and God rewarded them for their obedience (Daniel 3:1–30).

I have a personal story to show you how God was with us. Dylan and I just returned home from a trip to see relatives in North Carolina. I had a chiropractor appointment about fifteen minutes from my home. Before the appointment at 5:00 p.m., Dylan and I had some shopping to do. I was tired and in desperate need of an adjustment, as my back was bothering me. We took the highway to my appointment after many stops running errands. We sailed through two green lights and came upon the third, which was red. My son said, "Mom, it's red!" I went to brake and couldn't lift my foot to brake. Dylan tried frantically to pull the emergency brake with no luck. I went on the side of the road, still moving and coming upon the red light and intersection. Thank God the opposite direction traffic was not moving yet. I drove through the intersection and skimmed a dump truck on the passenger side of my car, finally hitting a pole that stopped us. Dylan said, "Mom, are you okay? I'm okay." I said, "Yes, but I can taste blood." As we waited for the emergency personnel, I realized I broke a tooth during the accident, and the blood was from the broken tooth. My chest hurt so badly, especially when I would breathe in. I went by ambulance, as it hurt and scared me to breathe. My husband came to the scene and took Dylan to meet me at the hospital. As the ambulance drove down the highway to the hospital, I realized I never made it to the chiropractor, which I desperately needed after getting hit hard during the accident.

I tell this story to say God's hand protected us. Dylan had only a bruised elbow, and I lost part of a tooth and was very sore from my seat belt. It was a miracle we weren't killed, especially Dylan because I sideswiped a dump truck on his side of the car that was waiting at the light at the intersection. God's hand watched over us. Dylan and I had just returned home from two weeks of visiting relatives while our bathroom was remodeled. I desperately wanted to be home, but as we left the hospital, my parents insisted we stay with them so I could recover. We stayed with them for two weeks. Thank God for them. I never experienced such pain in my chest area before. The seat belt did its job, but even simple movements became difficult. I took megadoses of ibuprofen to function. We moved back home two weeks before school was to start. I finally got to use our new bathroom that was remodeled because our old bathroom was in dire need of repair.

The car I drove in the accident was a Honda CRV. It was like a tank, enduring the accident. My car was totaled; however, we were not totaled. When I realized how the Honda protected us in the crash, I purchased another Honda CRV. I went six weeks without a car, which was not easy. My husband drove us to doctors' appointments, grocery shopping, church, etc. I did not realize all the places we went until we had to be taken everywhere and depended on someone else to drive us to and fro. I was so happy and scared at the same time when my car came in and I could drive again. I was waiting on God to get the confidence to get behind the wheel. By God's grace, I have been enabled to go through every challenge. I named my last Honda Gracie, and now after our accident, my new Honda is Gracie II. I have named my last three to four cars, as I am certain God allows me to function and meet every hurdle with a positive attitude. Listening to criticism after the accident was challenging. I never wanted to be the center of attention. Suddenly, I had to listen to critiques of my driving ability. Fear tried to get a hold of me and Dylan too. Remember, fear is not from God. I had to face my fear and get on the horse again (drive again). The first time I drove in six weeks was to drive my new car home from the dealership. I had much pressure from my family to get hand controls in my new car.

Honda has a mobility program that paid for hand controls to be purchased and installed in my new car. I was always opposed to hand controls, but what a blessing they have turned out to be. After the accident, fear plagued Dylan about riding with me. The hand controls have allowed me to feel safer driving. You can still drive normally using the brake, or, if tired, you can use the hand brake as a backup. I did not understand how the hand controls worked. They seemed like an unknown burden with a handicapped label for all the world to know and judge. Honestly, anyone can drive my car normally without having to ever use the hand controls. What a blessing they are. It is comforting to feel secure having a backup if you need to use them. For a time, Dylan would tell me how to drive. He was jumpy as I drove, and I finally did tell him that he must trust that God would protect us.

Remember, if you need hand controls in your car, they are a blessing until your healing manifests. Appreciate every day. I know God did not cause our accident, but he surely was there with us in it. I still believe despite all I have gone through, God will use hard times to mold us for the good. Today, Dylan and I ride together. Other than him being a know-it-all sixteen-year-old teenager, we drive without fear. He tells me how to drive and controls the radio, which honestly gets on my last nerve. I remind myself, "This age will pass." It is payback time. Three years have passed since the accident. Now, Dylan has his driver's license and I tell him how drive and I control the radio.

I do speak the Word of God in my car and over us. The Word of God is most powerful. I know ultimately God loves us, and he will protect us no matter what happens. "So is my Word that goes out from my mouth: It will not return to me empty, but will accomplish what I desire and achieve the purpose for which I sent it" (Isaiah 55:11).

Good news! God's Word will not return to him void. Speak positive words over your life and situation. In the back of this book, I have included healing scriptures that you should speak out of your mouth. God will perform what his Word says. Be careful not to speak negative words because words have power, and you will get what you speak, either positive or negative. Watch what you say because the Lord will do what he hears you say.

An example of this is our son in school. He had to take a foreign language in seventh and eighth grade. He chose French during sixth grade when the kids had to pick their first and second choices of language. He never liked his French teacher. She spoke very fast and was a bit scattered. She went from topic to topic, and Dylan would get lost trying to follow her. He struggled those two years. He constantly spoke negatively to me about French. I always told him that you get what you speak out of your mouth. I would quote to him Numbers 14:28, which states, "As surely as I live declares the Lord, I will do to you the very things I hear you say." You must watch what you say because you will get what you've spoken. Dylan finally passed once he believed he could succeed in French. Lots of prayers from his mom surely helped also.

Remember, God loves you and has an awesome plan for your life. You may be thinking, *I've done so much wrong in my life. God is my judge and won't forgive all my sins.* Yes, he will. God sent his own Son, Jesus, to die on the cross for our sins, and we can be redeemed by asking Jesus into our hearts. "For God so greatly loved and dearly prized the world that he gave up his only begotten Son, so that whoever believes in him shall not perish but have eternal (everlasting) life" (John 3:16–17, AMP).

God's Word says, "In a little burst of wrath I hid my face from you for a moment, but with age enduring love and kindness I will have compassion and mercy on you, says the Lord, your Redeemer" (Isaiah 54:8, AMP). The key is asking Jesus to come into your heart, and he will cleanse you and forgive all your sins. All God's promises in his Word are yours once you become a believer. An awesome book that I recently read is *The Purpose Driven Life* by Rick Warren. This inspirational book reveals to you why you were created and that God has a purpose and plan for your life. You are not a mistake. It is God's will that all people come to him and walk in his will for their lives. Until such a time, you will not feel complete in all you try to do in your life. You will have a void until you trust and turn to your Creator and allow him to take over. You will find real peace as you trust God to be the captain of your life.

Only Believe

One area the Lord has worked in me about is calling those things that are not as if they are already done. When you are in the middle of the sickness, it is not easy to say, "I am healed" while experiencing pain or symptoms. However, that is the way God's kingdom operates. We have to believe before we see it.

God has showed me numerous times during this illness to call things as I want them to be not as they actually are. (read Romans 4:16–21) It is not the easiest thing to do when you have a day in pain or are struggling to function in such a busy world. However, it is God's way to bring forth healing or whatever you are speaking out of your mouth and praying for. Remember, we get what we speak, be it good or bad, in our lives. In Numbers 14:28, God says, "As surely as I live, declares the Lord, I will do to you the very things I heard you say." When you know God's promises in his Word to you, you can claim them for yourself. Romans 8:24–25 speaks on hope. "But hope that is seen is no hope at all. Who hopes for what he already has? But if we hope for what we do not yet have, we wait for it patiently."

I have come to the place where I know in my spirit that I am healed, and my body has to line up with God's Word! It is much easier to speak positively out of my mouth, claiming his Word, knowing that is the way God will perform his work. I am walking by faith, not by sight (2 Corinthians 5:7). We must believe God's Word to be true. I have many family members and acquaintances that can't understand the joy in me. They see me struggle with my sickness and if they do not know Jesus, they are stumped how I can smile and be happy; they are walking by sight. Most of the time, I encourage whoever sees me with my positive attitude because I know the healing power of God is working in me. I often say to someone who asks me how I am with a pitiful attitude, "My heart is beating, and I am breathing—I have no complaints." Try speaking out loud, "The healing power of God is working in me mightily." A few years ago, Dylan and I stopped to pick up some lunch after church at a small gas station on the way to our cottage. Unbeknown to me, a lady was in the store who knew my dad and me. A few days later, my dad called me and said this woman ran into him and told him she thought his daughter was in the store on Sunday. She said, "She radiates. She looks so happy." I never even noticed the woman and never spoke a word to her. She saw the glow of the Lord and his joy in me. My circumstances do not cause me to be joyful or radiate; however, my relationship with the Lord Jesus does! I truly feel joyful in my heart and doing

God's will has become my primary focus. As time has gone on, I am now able to pray, "Not my will but yours be done." Once you get the focus off yourself and on God, your healing will manifest. Keep looking up!

In the midst of my struggles, I am peaceful and not worried about tomorrow. God's Word says, "Do not worry or be anxious about tomorrow, for tomorrow will have worries and anxieties of its own. Sufficient for each day is its own trouble" (Matthew 6:34, AMP). I am thankful we don't know the future prior to events that happen. On Mother's Day a few years ago, I became very embarrassed. I will explain. My family and I went out to dinner at a local restaurant near my hometown. Mother's Day is this restaurant's opening day for the summer, and the location is very popular for local families to enjoy Mother's Day dinner. I took my scooter in, and once I got in my seat at our table, Dylan moved my scooter out of the way. After dinner, we got ready to leave, and Dylan brought my scooter to me so I could get on it and leave. We were seated at a table in the middle of a large dining room. The restaurant was full with it seemed every family from our small town. I went to get up to leave, holding on to the table and the back of the chair next to mine. I often use my upper body strength to lift myself up. As I got up, the chair slid, and down I went on the floor in the middle of the dining room. My family quickly came to lift me up and helped me onto my scooter. There I was the center of attention, and I just wanted to crawl in a hole. As we were leaving, several people stopped me on my scooter to see if I was okay. I just wanted to get out of the restaurant and go home. I imagined all the talk about me and MS. By the time I got to the car, I was crying and did not want to talk about the embarrassment I was feeling.

Only the grace of God saw me through that moment. The next day, my niece had a tennis match at the high school in the same town. I picked Dylan up at school, and we went to the tennis match. It had to be that God allowed me to attend without fear because I never questioned whether we should go or not. Do you know how many people from the night before we saw at the match? I was on my scooter and held my head high with a smile on my face. I was not sore after the fall the night before and knew God enabled me to go forward when life seemed to throw me a curveball. I am not certain I would want to go through that ordeal again, but I know God is good, and he saw me through it.

As you grow in your personal relationship, God's Word will become so real to you. It is awesome to rest and have assurance, knowing God is in control of every circumstance. "Peace I leave with you; my peace I give you: I do not give to you as the world gives. Do not let your hearts be troubled and do not be afraid" (John 14:27).

The world sees MS or any chronic illness as an incurable disease, and your family may have a wheelchair in the back of their minds. If you don't have one or if you do, there's good news! "With men this is impossible, but with God all things are possible" (Matthew 19:26). I have learned this ordeal is making me more like Christ. As I have, you will meet resistance through negative people who have a pessimistic attitude toward you and your faith. Remember faith will put you over the top of this mountain (sickness). Negativity will keep you in the pit of despair. What you say with your mouth will come to pass. Continually speak healing and thank God for it. You will see the manifestation come to pass in your body in God's perfect timing. Remember to praise God during the wait. Praise brings breakthrough. "I will praise you, O Lord, with all my heart; I will tell of all you wonders" (Psalm 9:1). Praise the Lord as you wait for God's promises to be fulfilled. "Praise the Lord, O my soul and forget not all his benefits—who forgives all your sins and heals all your diseases" (Psalm 103:2–3). You do not need to pay for what Jesus already paid for on the cross. A friend once told me something I never forgot. Say you received a bill from a store, for example. You thought you had to go pay the bill, but you knew it was already paid for by someone else (a friend). Would you go pay it again? The same is true for your healing. You don't have to pay for what Jesus already paid for. Simply believe what he did for you and rest knowing he has an awesome plan in it all. Regardless of your current circumstances, believe God's Word is true and it will come to pass.

The Importance of Prayer

Prayer is an awesome privilege of the believer. Prayer is powerful. Prayers do not have to be spiritual sounding and long. They can be short and sweet, to the point. Talk to God and bring him all your petitions with thanksgiving. God cares about every detail of our lives. Prayer should become so normal for you and me that we seek him even in the small things. I pray about our son at school, including his grades, issues on the bus or at school with certain classmates, and any other issues affecting him there. I pray about my haircut appointments, what to wear daily, or anything and everything throughout each day. Have faith and believe God hears even our simple prayers.

> "Have faith in God," Jesus answered. "I tell you the truth, if anyone says to this mountain, 'Go, throw yourself into the sea,' and does not doubt in his heart but believes what he says will happen, it will be done for him. Therefore, I tell you whatever you

ask for in prayer, believe that you have received it, and it will be yours."

Mark 11:22–24

Remember, God wants us well. At the end of Mark 11:25 there is a stipulation. It says, "And when you stand praying, if you hold anything against anyone, forgive him, so that your Father in heaven may forgive you your sins." So we must search our heart to see if we have unforgiveness (a grudge) against anyone and forgive in order for God to answer our prayers.

Many times I have felt like my prayers were hitting the ceiling and bouncing right back to me, as if no one is hearing a word. Have you ever felt like that? Keep praying. God knows your heart, and he will answer your sincere prayer. "Do not be anxious about anything, but in everything by prayer and petition with thanksgiving present your requests to God" (Philippians 4:6).

When I realized I had to look inside myself as to anyone I had not forgiven over the years, I sat and made a list of whom I needed to forgive and what grudges I had been harboring in my heart. I wrote the names and what I was forgiving them for. This was not an easy task because I had to go back and remember all the past hurt. I prayed and told the Lord I forgave each one and then I tore up the list. There were many people I no longer see, so I wrote the list to clear my conscience and forgive as God's Word says we should so he will forgive us. Certainly, if someone is in your life that you need to forgive, you can tell him you forgive him for whatever it is that hurt you. One person the Lord has been dealing with me to forgive is my husband. I have been tested in this area. On June 13, 2005, my husband lost his job and therefore was home 24/7. His drinking became worse as he had far too much time on his hands. It is easier to endure his alcohol addiction when he was gone ten or more hours per day. I could handle the few hours at night until suddenly he was home cramping my style and peace. God gave me the grace to endure; however, one night during dinner Jeff got verbally abusive with our son. I could not take any more. His treatment was affecting Dylan, and I felt that was the straw that broke the camel's back for me. I made the decision Dylan and I would leave Jeff and move to my parents. We were with my parents for six weeks in February with snowy and cold weather, driving Dylan thirty minutes each way to and home from school. Finally, Jeff moved out so we could move back home. This was a very stressful time, but I knew I could no longer live in such an atmosphere of abuse for our son or myself.

Jeff and I were separated for nearly two years. I made the decision that Dylan and I would no longer live with alcohol. As I stated earlier, Jeff is an alcoholic, and I tried to be the wife like those in the Bible for so long turning the other cheek. I am not advocating separation; however, my situation got to a point where I could no longer tolerate his chemical addiction. I went to a Christian counselor who told me I was doing the right thing for Dylan and myself. My counselor explained to me that alcohol is an addiction that I cannot change. Until Jeff makes a decision to get help, I realized the situation is out of my control. However,

I decided I would not tolerate alcohol in our home any longer. The stress Dylan and I dealt with daily was unhealthy. I have had to forgive Jeff in my heart for his choices that kept him from our home, which has left Dylan to pick up many of the manly duties around our home. Jeff and I are not legally separated, and I have no plans for divorce. I believe Jeff will be delivered, and our marriage will be restored. I am trying to see him through God's eyes. We have him over for dinner occasionally, I do his laundry unto the Lord, and we try to keep things as normal as possible for Dylan on birthdays and holidays. I pray for him often, believing with God all things are possible. I try to remember to hate the sin, not the sinner. I missed my sober husband and the normal life I know we could share. When your husband is not there for you, God will be your husband. God is also a father to Dylan, as his father is very far removed. I think the hurt Dylan endures when his dad does not spend time with him bothers me beyond what I can express. I am trusting God to be there for Dylan and me. Alcohol addiction is a real disease. The worst part is the alcoholic is in denial and does not believe he has a problem. I pray constantly for the blinders to come off Jeff's eyes so he will realize how his disease has affected his family. Separating the person from the disease is difficult because I think it is his choice to drink. I finally recognize that Jeff is way beyond his choice. He is at the point where his body cannot function without alcohol. I sometimes have to forgive Jeff daily to the Lord. This is in no way easy, but God has sustained us through this time. I continue to pray, believing God hears me and is working this out for our good.

When I realized unforgiveness could hinder my prayers, it was easier to dig deep and see any unforgiveness. "For if you forgive men when they sin against you, your heavenly Father will also forgive you. But if you don't forgive men their sins, your Father will not forgive your sins" (Matthew 6:14–15).

Jesus spoke about prayer while he was on the earth. Matthew 6:8 says,

> When you pray go into your room, close the door and pray to your Father, who is unseen, then your Father who sees what is done in secret will reward you. And when you pray do not keep on babbling like pagans, for they think they will be heard because of their many words. Do not be like them, for your Father knows what you need before you ask him.

This scripture reminds me of the religions that repeat the same prayers over and over again. Talk to God and tell him all that concerns you. Be real with God. He already knows our lives. You might be thinking, *Why should I bother praying?* Prayer is the key to unlock the blessings God has for you and me.

Walking through any illness, MS or another, can be so trying and can cause added stress to life. Know God is in control and start praying simply believing prayers and watch God bless you and your life. An essential part of successful prayers includes praying for others. In the story of Job, he was delivered when he prayed for his friends. In Job 42:10, the Word says, "Job prayed for his friends, the Lord made him prosperous again and gave him twice as much as he had before." As I pray, I remember my friends and family in need of salvation and healing. I pray for them before myself. When you are facing trouble or sickness yourself, the way to victory is to get your eyes off yourself and pray for others. It is vital to your emotional health and physical well-being each day to think of someone else and pray for him or her before yourself. My walk has been an awesome learning experience. I never knew before about the healing available to me through Jesus. I would not change what I have gone through, even as hard as it has been, to know a personal Savior and his awesome work on the cross for you and me.

"Therefore do not worry about tomorrow, for tomorrow will worry about itself. Each day has enough trouble of its own" (Matthew 6:34). Remember to always be thankful to the Lord. Don't just come to him in prayer asking, but always be thankful for all he has done and will do for you. Praise God during the wait for who he is and what he has already done on cross.

Always give thanks to the Lord and thank him even before you see the answers to your prayers. God's way is to call those things that are not as though they are already done. Pray always to the Lord. In James 4:2, it states, "You do not have, because you do not ask God." So keep asking in prayer. We have not because we ask not. Always ask in faith. Another awesome promise from the Word of God is found in Matthew 18:19–20: "Again, I tell you that if two of you on earth agree about anything you ask for, it will be done for you by my Father in heaven. For where two or three come together in my name, there I am with them." If you have a friend who stands in agreement with you for your healing or whatever your request may be, his Word tells us it will be done by our Father in heaven. Find a trusted Christian friend who you know will pray for you and agree with you for what you are asking. Be sure the person you pray with stands in agreement, believes as you do, and the prayer will be answered. God's Word works. A few months ago, I asked my pastor and a trusted friend at church to stand in agreement with me and pray for our son, Dylan. He was having trouble hearing. I took him to the ear doctor and found out he only had 30 percent hearing and needed surgery. A week before surgery was scheduled, I had him prayed for at church. The next day, he could hear 100 percent better. I waited four days and took him to the ear doctor the day before his scheduled surgery. Praise God, his surgery was canceled. His ears were clear, and he no longer required surgery. The doctor was amazed and told Dylan, "I guess you are going to school tomorrow and not the hospital." This miracle increased both my family's and my faith. God is so good.

Another Praise Report: Answered Prayer

In June 2002, I went to my yearly neurologist appointment. I, of course, prayed for a positive, encouraging appointment. I asked all my Christian friends, including my pastor, to pray for me. It is wonderful to have a church family of believers in Christ to lift you up in prayer when in need. They all agreed with me in praying and believed for a good report. At my appointment, my neurologist first talked to me to see what's been going on, as it had been a year since I had seen her. I told her that I stopped Copaxone in October 2001, and I was taking natural amino acids. She was disturbed and a bit negative that I was doing natural supplements. I told her I was seeing a chiropractor who treated patients with corrective care to fix the problem in the spine. I further explained I was in traction to correct my six subluxations (six places where my spine was out of proper alignment).

She informed me she did not believe in chiropractors. How unfortunate that a physician was so close-minded to the truth, particularly with MS. If your spine is misaligned, it directly affects the nervous system. Between the spinal bones, called vertebrae, are nerves that transport messages from the brain to all organs, tissues, and cells in the body. When a spinal vertebrae is out of alignment, it may put damaging pressure on the spinal nerves, causing interruptions to the vital nerve flow in the body. How could a neurologist not believe in chiropractic care? Needless to say, my appointment was off to a negative start.

She continued my exam and found everything the same as last year. She requested that I have another brain MRI to be sure there was no progression. I agreed and scheduled my MRI for three weeks later. I was very unnerved as I left my appointment. My doctor was so negative and put out with my positive outlook. I kept my eyes on the Lord and his promise in his Word. "By his wounds, you have been healed" (1 Peter 2:24). During my MRI, I prayed the entire time in the Spirit with my mind. Dr. Mihia told me she would call me with the results. I waited two and a half weeks for her phone call. I was very peaceful and let go of worrying about the results.

My son and I were in town doing errands one day (we were living at our cottage, as it was summer), and we stopped at home. There was a message on my answering machine. It was Dr. Mihia. Here is what she said, "I am very surprised but pleased. You have no enhancing lesions, as to say no activity, no active disease, at this time." Praise God! She went on to say she would see me at my next appointment (which was in one year), and I should bring my old and new MRI films so she could compare them. She told me to enjoy my summer.

It could not have been an easy phone call to make, as she expected a worsening of MS. She did not know my God and the healing power available to every believer. You can imagine how overjoyed I was, along with my family and friends, with this news. Now my body has to line up with the Word of God. You cannot go by feelings. You must stand on God's promises found in the Word of God, and your faith will make you whole. In Hebrews 11:1, the Scripture explains faith: "Now faith is being sure of what we hope for and certain of what we do not see."

Through my walk (illness), I have had much doubt from my husband, family, and friends, both saved and unsaved. I have continually, even on the hard days, said, "By his wounds I have been healed" (1 Peter 2:24). I had to remind myself that I am walking by faith. However, the doubters are walking by sight. In God's Word, it says in 2 Corinthians 4:18, "So we fix our eyes not on what is seen but on what is unseen."

Stand on God's Word even when it seems darkest and hopeless. Remember God's Word will not return to him void. Isaiah 55:11 states, "So shall my Word be that goeth forth out of my mouth; it shall not return to me void, but it shall accomplish that which I please, and it shall prosper in the thing for where to I sent it" (KJV). How reassuring! God's Word will do what it says. You don't have to remain sick. Jesus promised us divine health when he carried away our sins and sicknesses on the cross. If you have a waiting time as I have had, God will transform you into the image of his Son. Do not be discouraged by delay.

Do not go by how you feel on the outside. Healing from God begins on the inside (in your spirit). While waiting on the physical manifestation of my healing, every time I have blood work, my results are always perfect. Yet symptoms still linger. I have to remind myself of these principles. I am healed; my insides confirm it every time I have testing done, including an MRI. God revealed to me that healing comes from the inside out. Feed your spirit God's Word by meditating on and speaking out loud healing scriptures (see the back of this book). The Lord always begins on the inside. You can know things on the inside that you don't see or feel yet on the outside. But because you know it in your spirit, believe it and say it out of your mouth. It will surely come to pass. In John 15:7, God's Word says, "If you remain in me and my words remain in you, ask whatever you wish, and it will be given you."

My father bought me a plaque from a trip to Arizona. I found it to be very encouraging.

Don't Quit

When things go wrong as they sometimes will
when the road you're trudging seems all up hill.
When you are feeling low and the stress is high,
and you want to smile but have to sigh.
When worries are getting you down a bit…
by all means pray and don't you quit.
Success is failure turned inside out.
God's hidden gift in the clouds of doubt.
You can never tell how close you are—
it may be near when it seems so far.
So trust in the Lord when you're hardest hit.
It is when things go wrong that you must not quit.

To Walk in Divine Health, You Must Walk in Love

This is an area in which the Lord has been speaking to me about for some time. We cannot expect to walk in divine health and not be walking in love toward others. You see, God is love. "Dear friends, let us love one another, for love comes from God. Everyone who loves has been born of God and knows God. Whoever does not love, does not know God, because God is love" (1 John 4:7–8). God sent his only Son, Jesus, to die on the cross for all sinners. He loved us so much while we were still sinners, and, therefore, he gave a new commandment. Jesus says, "A new command I give you: Love one another as I have loved you, so you must love one another" (John 13:34). The God kind of love is not the same as natural human love. Natural human love can turn to hatred overnight, but God's love never fails. The God kind of love is unconditional. There is nothing you can do or need to do to earn God's love. He showed the ultimate sacrifice by dying on the cross for your sins and mine. Just receive his love by accepting his Son's loving sacrifice.

Honestly, I am very compassionate and loving to others, but when it came to my own household, my marriage, I have struggled in this area. My husband can be the hardest person for me to show love to, particularly once I have been hurt by his words or actions. You see, when my husband drinks alcohol, his personality changes, and many times he says very hurtful things to me. During my illness, the last thing I want or need is stress from him. After a long time, I finally realized we must show love unto the Lord because of what he did for us on the cross. You may think the person who hurt you deserves to be treated improperly, and your flesh wants to retaliate, getting him or her back for your hurt. However, that is not God's way. We need to forgive the person and trust God to handle the matter. Speaking from personal experience, I would always tell about the hurt I experienced. I finally realized if I paid no attention to a suffered wrong, God could handle the matter much better than I could. We have to trust that God is our vindicator, and if we take our hands off the situation, God can work. This is not easy, but with time and persistence, doing it God's way will allow you to have peace, no matter what storms come. I used the following scripture to get me through the times when it seemed unbearable. In addition, I had to remember God is in control not me. God has a plan and purpose for out lives as believers—only believe and trust his goodness.

First Corinthians 13:4–8 states,

> Love endures long and is patient and kind; love never is envious nor boils over with jealousy, is not boastful or vainglorious, does not display itself haughtily. It is not conceited, it is not rude and does not act unbecomingly. Love (God's love in us) does not insist on its own rights or its own way, for it is not self seeking; it is not touchy or fretful or resentful; it takes no account of the evil done to it (it pays no attention to a suffered wrong). It does not rejoice at injustice and unrighteousness but rejoices when right and truth prevail. Love bears up under anything and everything that comes, is ever ready to believe the best of every person, its hopes are fadeless under all circumstances and it endures everything (without weakening). Love never fails (never fades out or becomes obsolete or comes to an end.)
>
> (AMP)

Let this scripture soak into your minds and hearts. The Word of God covers all aspects of relationships that we all encounter in our daily lives. Sometimes a wife or husband suffers and puts up with things, but he or she is not too kind while enduring. I myself am guilty of this. However, the God kind of love endures long and is patient and kind while it endures.

God's love doesn't weaken, fade out, or come to an end. It never fails. Although we are separated, I know God is in this situation. As I stated earlier, wisdom told me when I could no longer tolerate what the alcohol was doing to our family. I believe God will honor my commitment to our marriage despite the bump in the road we are now enduring.

I think about how God loved me through all the sinful days and years. I am so thankful he is a patient God and waited for me to ask Jesus to abide in me and take over my life. How awesome! I, in turn, am praying for me to be patient with my husband, knowing Jeff will see victory, and our marriage will be restored.

When dealing in a relationship that seems hard and difficult, look at the previous scripture, 1 Corinthians 13. Remember how much God put up with in our lives before we were saved, and yet he welcomes us with open arms.

There are times when I have to say to myself, "Pay no attention to a suffered wrong and take no account of an evil done to you." It may be in a store while shopping and someone will be rude, and I will tell him or her, "Have a blessed day" or "God bless you." You will notice as you walk in love consistently, there are many people in this world that are angry and unhappy. I know when someone is nasty toward me, there is something in his or her life causing his or her anger. If we can learn to look at all these people through Jesus eyes, (how he sees them) your whole perspective changes. I often pray that God will let me see others and my husband through his (God's) eyes. Not to mention that when you walk through sickness, you become very humble and appreciate being in a store versus unable to go shopping at all. In the past, I can remember times I was shopping on the store scooter or my own scooter. Many people are in a hurry and rude. However, I am experiencing the joy of the Lord and thankful I can drive to the store to go shopping. The automatic carts are a blessing and allow you to shop without getting exhausted from your shopping trip. Thank God they are available until God removes the need to use one in your life. Remember, people without a personal Savior, Jesus, are part of a lost and dying world. Those without Jesus have no hope and are living in darkness. The truth is they fear death because they do not know that they can spend eternity in heaven. I am amazed at the numerous fears many people live with. We need to cast our cares and fears on him. First Peter 4:7 states, "Cast all your anxiety on him because he cares for you." As I wrote earlier, I have no fear of MS getting worse or dying. I used to be full of fear before my salvation, but now I know a loving father God who has my best interest in mind. God's Word says in Jeremiah 29:11, "For I know the thoughts and plans I have for you, says the Lord, thoughts and plans for welfare and peace and not for evil, to give you hope in your final outcome" (AMP).

When you fail to walk in love, you open the door for evil (Satan) in your life. Exodus 23:25–26 says, "Ye shall serve the Lord your God, and he shall bless thy bread, and thy water; and I will take sickness away from the midst of thee. There shall nothing cast their young, nor be barren, in thy land; the number of thy days I will fulfill" (KJV). You can translate these verses in this way. Keep my commandment of love and I will take sickness from the midst of you, and the number of your days I will fulfill.

You see, if you are not walking in love, all that Jesus died for, which includes healing, will not work for you. When you are a Christian, you are protected from evil if you walk in love. When you are born-again, God himself will write the new commandment of love or the new law of the God kind of love in our hearts and spirits. The love of God is shed abroad in our hearts by the Holy Ghost, which is given unto us as Christians. You see, if the law of love is written in your heart and you are walking in the light of God's love, you are not going to break any of the Ten Commandments. In the Old Testament, the Ten Commandments were given to curb sin. But if you are walking in love, you are not going to break any of the Ten Commandments.

How awesome! When you are born again by asking Jesus into your heart, the love of God is in you. You are a new creature. Second Corinthians 5:17 says, "Therefore, if anyone be in Christ, he is a new creation: the old has gone, the new has come." If you fail to walk in love, you open the door of your life and body to the devil (Satan).

The devil is real. You may be thinking, *I don't want the devil bothering me, so I don't want to be a born-again Christian.* Guess what? The devil has full reign over your life if you chose to reject asking Jesus into your life. Hell is a real place, and there you will spend eternity apart from God. Satan is the author of sickness, not God. God is the healer. If you want to walk in divine health and enjoy life to the fullest, spending eternity in heaven versus hell, don't waste another day trying to live this life apart from Jesus. His Word says in John 10:10b, "I have come that they might have life and have it to the full." I have seen many relatives and friends who are not Christians have terminal cancer and die premature deaths. They don't know a personal Savior and have no hope.

I am so grieved to stand back and watch as Satan is destroying them. I have, of course, told them about Jesus and salvation. Some have accepted the invitation to ask Jesus to take over their lives while others haven't. One of my aunts asked Jesus into her heart when she became sick. She died of cancer three weeks later. God took her home the day before Easter ten years ago. I am so thankful she said the salvation prayer prior to her death. I know she is in heaven now for eternity, and God took her home quickly. The devil put cancer on her, but she was saved from long-suffering. It was not God's will for her to die so young. She was precious, and I miss her so much. You see, Satan is real, and without Jesus at the helm of your life, Satan can and may put sickness or disease upon you. When you are a child of God, he (God) is in control. He knows best. "I am the Lord your God who teaches you what is best for you, who directs you in the way you should go" (Isaiah 48:17). I am so thankful I can trust a loving God, and I am not in control because I would have it all messed up. God will work every circumstance of your life, including sickness, for your good if you trust him. God's Word says, "And we know that in all things God works for the good of those who love him, who are called according to his purpose" (Romans 8:28).

From this day forward, commit to walking in love. If you get into unforgiveness or lack of love toward another, just repent. God is a good God. There are times when we all fail and say or do things that we know are wrong and get out of walking in love. Take God at his Word. God said, "If we confess our sins, he is faithful and just and will forgive us our sins and to purify us from all unrighteousness" (1 John 1:9). I still have to sometimes repent daily. Life is not always easy, but God knows best and is working in me mightily. Remember the saying, "Father knows best." Thank God he loves us and is patient with us.

An awesome privilege of being a child of God is if you know you are walking in love and Satan attacks you, your children, or your home, you can boldly say, "Satan, take your hands off me (or whatever he is trying to affect) because I am walking in love." Failing to walk in the God kind of love can affect every area of your life, including your health. I've determined to walk in love whether anyone else does or not. Remember, you do not know anyone's life unless you hop into their life. Many people have deep hurts, and they do not feel loved. I know my husband has deep hurts, as he was sent to military school at a young age. He has deep wounds from that experience. He was not allowed to grow up in his home with his parents and siblings. I believe he did not feel loved and buried the hurt and started drinking alcohol beginning many years ago. Always think about the fact that someone who seems unhappy or unloving may have a past that is tormenting them. You will have less stress if you exhibit God's love. The reward is the joy of the Lord will absolutely be your strength.

A friend once told me something as I was complaining about my husband that I have never forgotten. She said, "If you love him, God will change him. If you try to change him, God will love him."

The Promises of God Must Be Birthed

As I am about to complete this book, I have come to realize that waiting on a promise such as divine healing is like birthing a baby. Once you come to know and understand the promises in God's Word for the believer, you claim the promise, standing and believing until you see and feel the manifestation.

About seven years ago, I had a desire to write a book about my experience with MS and the journey I have traveled. I thought I would write when I was on the other side of this struggle (or fire, as I have called it in this book). At a Wednesday night service at church, a dear sister in the Lord told me the following. Sister Gwen Dailey gave the sermon that Wednesday evening, which was most powerful. She explained that we all have a baby on the inside of us that needs to be birthed. Over time, we forgot or buried our baby inside us. The baby she was speaking of is a promise from God's Word. She had an altar call at the end of service for those who wanted their vision (baby) to be revealed to them. I went up to the altar not sure what the baby (vision) inside me was, and I wanted to know. Sister Gwen came to me and immediately she said, "You need to write." I suddenly remembered the desire I had of writing a book, but I planned to write it when I was totally on the other side of this illness. Sister Gwen said, "You need to write it now."

I started this book a few days later. As I near closure writing this book, I am in the birthing process. With a pregnancy, the baby is born in God's perfect timing. The same is true with one of God's promises; it will happen in his (God's) perfect timing, but you must believe during the wait that it will come to pass. Just as with pregnancy, you eat right, take your vitamins, and prepare a room for your new arrival. Also, you do everything to be comfortable while you wait, such as maternity clothes and anything necessary to sustain you during this, for many, uncomfortable time. The same is true with any items you may use to help you during your illness time. I wrote earlier about my scooter, my cane, my use of automatic carts in stores, and my hand controls in my car, to name a few. I never wanted any of these items. I can now say that these items are a help and a true blessing. I think I believed using help was giving into MS. However, I now realize it is okay to use the necessary help to assist you while you wait for God's promises to be manifested in your life. Recently. my father ordered me Link to Life as my parents were traveling to Arizona for a month. They wanted to know I could press a button if I had a physical need, and I would have help come to my aid. It is not a lack of faith to use assistance to get through each day without struggle. With a promise from God's Word, you feed on the Word of God, believe his Word will come to pass, and prepare for the manifestation (arrival) while waiting like you already have it. This book has been my preparing for the birth of God's promise. Recently, my pastor said to me, "You are in labor, you are dilating, and you need to push." Honestly, as time has gone on, it feels like labor. I pushed for so long while in labor for our son, I did not think his head was ever coming out. As time lingers while waiting on a promise from God, remember God's timetable is not our timetable. He is in control and knows best. In Isaiah 55:8–9, God's Word says, "For my thoughts are not your thoughts, neither are your ways my ways. As the heavens are higher than the earth, so are my ways higher than your ways and my thoughts higher than your thoughts."

Just as childbirth makes us weary, I am weary in the wait; however, I know God's Word will not return void. Isaiah 55:11 states, "So is my word that goes out from my mouth: it will not return to me empty, but will accomplish what I desire and achieve the purpose for which I sent it." Great news! God will not be late; his timing is perfect. Read the story of Abraham and Sarah in the book of Genesis in the Bible. They waited for God's promise of a child to be fulfilled. Abraham praised God during the wait, and he believed God's Word to him that he would be the father of many nations. It did come to pass in God's perfect timing. Also in Genesis, Noah had to wait years while building a boat during a drought. When the rains came, he and his family survived because he was obedient to the Lord by building a boat when it had not rained for many years.

Others may think you are crazy when it looks like nothing is happening, but you are taking God at his Word. This can be especially difficult for family members who are unsaved. They only see struggle. It seems like no one believes like I believe. They have sincere concern watching their loved one believing and trusting that God's Word will come to pass. Don't let their doubt discourage you and your walk with God. You will get discouraged if you buy into the negative. I have dealt with my share of negative comments. Your family and friends may think you have lost your mind believing, for them, what seems like denial of reality. I do not deny the facts, but God's Word is greater than the facts. I often pray for the manifestation so God will allow others to see what I have been believing for so long. If you are believing God's promises and are awaiting the manifestation, do not lose heart. It will come to pass; only believe. In the interim, God's grace is sufficient for every day. The devil will put negative thoughts in your mind to make you think it will always be this way and it will never come to pass. The devil is a liar. Rest in what God has said in his Word in Exodus 33:14: "My presence will go with you and I will give you rest." The thing you are believing for will come to pass. Stay in the Word of God. His Word brings life and light. In Habakkuk 2:3, God's Word states, "For the revelation awaits an appointed time; it speaks of the end and will not prove false. Though it linger, wait for it. It will certainly come and will not delay." Your promise will certainly come even though the time may seem to linger. God's timing is perfect. Remember to praise God right where you are. Praise brings breakthrough. Get your eyes off your circumstances and on Jesus. In Jeremiah 1:2, God's Word states, "Before I formed you in the womb, I knew you. Before you were born I set you apart." God knew you before he placed you in your mother's womb. How incredibly awesome! He approved of us and had a plan for our lives before we were even born.

I recently had revelation that this battle (sickness) belongs to the Lord. I started thinking how I am his child, bought and paid for with a price, and he has defeated the enemy on the cross. Anything we go through as a Christian is orchestrated and approved from the throne of God before it can affect us. Lately, I have felt like I am under constant attack from the enemy. However, I know God is allowing the trials that have affected me. I in no way mean to say enduring trials is easy. They can be very hard and uncomfortable. This wait has been difficult, but God's grace has allowed me to endure every trial. When I reflect back as I write about many of the struggles I have gone through, I remind myself that I have gone through them all. If I did not know Jesus, I hate to think where I would be. I suppose I would give up and look at this illness as the world does. Thank God I no longer have that old pessimistic and negative attitude. You don't have to live that way either. In the midst, I keep praising the Lord, knowing victory is just around the corner. "But as for me I will always have hope; I will praise you more and more" (Psalm 71:14). When you realize who you are in Christ, it becomes easier to let go and let God. Trust is a big issue. We must trust that God is a good God and will not allow more than we can handle to come upon us. He always has our best interest in mind. Your breakthrough is on the horizon. Speak the result you desire out of your mouth.

Remember, we get what we speak, either positive or negative. In Joel 3:10, God's Word says, "Let the weak say, I am strong." Even if you do not feel strong, begin speaking, "I am strong" out of your mouth. Just as it is with our salvation, we speak with our mouth and believe in our heart that Jesus is Lord over our lives. You don't have to do another thing to be born again. You will find you will be changed gradually. The same is true concerning healing. Speak the desired result out of your mouth. Your healing will come to pass; just believe you receive. Read Mark 11:22–24. We cannot go by feelings. Continually speak to your body. "I am not moved by what I see. I am not moved by what I feel. I call my body this way. My body is whole and strong. I call it no other way; I am well. By Jesus's wounds, I am healed and that settles the issue." God says in Numbers 14:28, "As surely as I live, declares the Lord, I will do to you the very things I heard you say." Be careful what you are saying. Only say what you want to manifest in your body and life. There are no drive-through breakthroughs in the kingdom of God. I have been totally changed through this fire (sickness). If I received the manifestation instantly, I would not have experienced the trials and suffering that have transformed my life for the good. Your attitude during the trial will determine you altitude. In James 1:2–3, God's Word states,

"Consider it pure joy, my brothers, whenever you face trials of many kinds because you know that the testing of your faith develops perseverance." We are to be joyful no matter what we are going through. It will produce patience in us to endure while waiting on God. Ask God for wisdom as you go through the trial or sickness. I can admit I have not always been patient and questioned God why many things have happened to me. I have wondered what I did to deserve such torment. I remind myself that God has a plan in it all. I recently read a book entitled *God Meant It For Good* by R.T. Kendall, which is a look at the life of Joseph in the Bible. What a wonderful book that explains how God allowed Joseph to go through much hardship in preparation for his victory in the end. As a child of God's, he works all things together for our good. In Romans 8:28, God says, "And we know that in all things God works for the good of those who love him, who have been called according to his purpose." All things that happen to us may not seem good at the time; however, God uses each circumstance for our good and his purpose for us. God has a plan for your life that is far greater than anything you can conceive.

It has been a comfort to me during my intense trials to know God is on the throne, approving of all I have gone through, and he will bring me out of this as I belong to him. I know he has a good plan for my life. This is not to say it has been easy during the trial but far from it. I will give you an example. I have fallen several times in my home during my disability. Almost each time I had been in the Word of God either reading, watching a tape, or listening to healing scriptures. When it happens, it is like someone shoves me and down I go. Afterward, I have learned to praise God. I say, "You have gotten me through every time this has happened before." It is totally God that I have not broken any bones, and I am not really sore the next day. It is like the angels place me on the floor even though I hit hard. Although I do not understand it all, I know the one (Jesus) who has it under control, and victory is mine. You will succeed in your labor and delivery of God's promise. A scripture that allowed me to rest on God's perfect timing is in Acts 1:7: "Jesus said it is not for you to know the times or dates the Father has set by his own authority." Keep looking up, and he will see you through to the finish line. A friend of mine gave me the following poem:

In God's Time

I wait on God to bring to pass
all that he has promised me,
And as I wait I rest in faith in what I cannot see.
For in his way he will pro-
vide at just the perfect time.
Everything that's good and right
to bless this life of mine.

Laughter Is the Best Medicine

God's Word says in Proverbs 17:22, "A cheerful heart is good medicine, but a crushed spirit dries up the bones." The Good News Bible states, "Being cheerful keeps you healthy." I would like to share some funny stories that I made a decision to laugh about and enjoy the moment versus crying or being embarrassed, knowing God had a good plan through it all.

Take a moment and laugh with me. Many of these times, I felt like I was on display, but God used them for his glory.

In September 2003, our son, Dylan, was starting a new school. He was going into the fifth grade and changing from an elementary school to an intermediate school. In late August, 2003, the school was opened so students and parents could take self-guided tours to find their classrooms. Some of the teachers were available to meet the children also. My good friend Susan went with us, as her son Chris was in the same grade. We parked in the back parking lot. It was quite a distance to walk to their new classrooms. I used my cane, and Susan helped me. After walking a while, I needed to sit and rest. Susan took the boys to find their classrooms while I rested. While sitting, I noticed a utility cart in front of me. I had been sitting in a classroom chair. Susan came back with the boys to get me and I thought how the chair I was sitting on could be placed on the utility cart, and she could push me. I knew this would save my energy. . What a good friend. She pushed me to each classroom, and I even met some teachers sitting like a queen on the bulky cart. It was hard for Susan to push as it steered crooked because of the size. How we laughed. Talk about humbling. I met two of my son's new teachers riding on the chariot (utility cart) that God provided. She pushed me right in the rooms on this bulky utility cart, and there I sat higher up than everyone else. I even met the principal and other staff sitting on my perch. Needless to say, I did not have my scooter yet. What a blessing my scooter has turned out to be. We made a fun time out of what could have been an embarrassing time for me. We definitely made a memory in the new school. Dylan and I still laugh about it today. God provided a way to save my energy and allowed me to still see his new school with him.

My brother got married the next month, and his reception was at a golf course. The tables were set up in a pavilion that was used to store golf carts when they were not used for parties. The bathroom for guests was in a different building, and after dinner, my sister asked me if I had to go to the bathroom. She helped me, and I used my cane to go outside to get a golf cart to ride to the other building. Remember, I did not yet buy a scooter. She drove me to the bathroom and then back to the reception. When we got back to the reception, she drove right into the reception hall with me on the golf cart. Nothing like making a grand entrance! She drove right up to a table where a bunch of my family was sitting. Everyone roared with laughter. We had to wait to get off the golf cart so many could take pictures of us. There again, I made another memory.

Another time, I went grocery shopping to a local store. Those automatic carts are a blessing, but this particular day, I wasn't so sure. I went around the store doing my shopping, and my cart was very full. I turned down the soda pop aisle to get mineral water when the motor of the automatic scooter died right in front of the Coke and Pepsi. I never even drink soda, and there I was stuck in the soda aisle. There was not a person in sight to ask for store help. My cane was in the car, so there I sat waiting for a person to ask for help. I was almost done shopping, and I just wanted to get my water and go home. We can be in a hurry even on an automatic cart. Finally, a lady came to the opposite end of the aisle, so I yelled to her to find a grocery store employee who could help me. She found an employee who went to the office to get me assistance. A man that worked at the store came and asked me to get off the scooter. He pushed a button in the back and then the scooter worked fine. Once again, I was on display. I resumed my shopping and proceeded to the checkout. I was flustered at what seemed like an eternity sitting in the soda pop aisle, but I now realize patience was being worked out in me.

Finally, I ordered a scooter. I waited a long time to get one, but I am so glad I finally made the decision to buy one, as it saves my energy and gives me freedom. The scooter is foldable and portable. It was a blessing because it is easy to take in and out of the car. Our son, Dylan, is so good at taking it in and out of the car that it takes him less than a minute. I know you may be like me when I did not want to give in to using a scooter, but remember God's Word is true, and it will come to pass. As I stated earlier, it is not a lack of faith to use necessary help that will make your life easier during the wait. A friend told me a story that helped me realize I should use whatever God provides. A man was in a flood where he lived. As the water rose, he went onto his roof. Two separate times someone came by in a boat to rescue him. The man refused to go with the rescue men and told both men that he was waiting for God to save him. Using necessary help does not mean you are giving up. I believe it is smart and most humbling to use whatever makes life easier. You will be so glad when you obtain needed assistance and wonder why you waited so long. Just because you use assistance during the wait does not mean he will not bring his healing promise to pass in your life. In Isaiah 43:13, God says, "No one can deliver out of my hand. When I act, who can reverse it?"

Our son played soccer in the spring one year after I got the scooter. My husband and I went to all his games, and I used the scooter, as it was a long walk to most of the soccer fields. One Sunday afternoon, we went to a game at a school about half an hour away from our home. It was near my hometown. I got on the scooter in the parking lot to go to the field. I did not use a little ramp to get up on the sidewalk. My husband, Dylan, and I went down the parking lot further to what looked like another ramp but turned out to be uneven ground with broken concrete. I wasn't sure if I should take my scooter up it, but my husband said, "Go for it," so I did. Guess what? I flipped the scooter on its side with me on it. Several parents and kids were walking to the soccer field. About five men and my husband rushed over to pick the scooter with me on it upright. I was embarrassed and shocked it happened. My parents and sister came to the game to watch Dylan play. Frankly, I wanted to crawl in a hole and forget about what happened to me on my scooter. Jeff proceeded to tell my family the whole story. Other parents around him could hear him tell the story. I was totally humiliated. I have been so humbled through it all. Being humble is not a bad thing. Actually, God wants us to be humble, not full of pride. His Word says in Proverbs 29:23, "Pride lands me flat on my face but humility prepares me for honor" (Message Bible). I laugh about it now; however, at the time, I was not laughing.

Dylan and I went on vacation one summer to North Carolina. We have an aunt and four cousins who live there. A few of us went to Myrtle Beach. We made some funny memories. Two of my cousins, Kris and Kim, helped me to the beach. I took the scooter across a grass section near a sand dune. We tried to figure out how I could go over the sand dune easily. Kris tried to give me a piggyback ride, but we both landed on the ground, laughing hysterically. Then Kris and Kim decided to carry me with my arms around their necks, and they lifted me up under my butt. They carried me like a queen. One guy asked Kris as they walked swiftly past carrying me, "What is wrong with her?" Kris responded, "Oh, nothing. She is just lazy." We cracked up laughing. We got out to the water and sat in low chairs right in the water. After a while, many went up to the pool. As I sat there enjoying the ocean view, the tide was coming in. Dylan was body surfing, and I yelled for him to go get someone to move me, all the chairs, and stuff back out of the surf. By the time someone came, I had water up to my neck, trying to hold onto the three chairs and all the clothes and beach stuff so they wouldn't float away. I thought I was going out to sea. Kim finally came to move the chairs, all the stuff and me back out of the surf. She was hysterically laughing.

While we were moving back, a lifeguard came up to us and asked if we needed help. The lifeguard went on to tell us they have a beach wheelchair. Kim and I looked at each other like, "You have to be kidding." Who knew they made such a thing? Kim went to the lifeguard afterward and reserved one for the next day. The next morning, she went to the lifeguard stand and picked it up. Oh my, have you ever seen one of them? It was made out of PVC with huge tires that floated. Kim pushed it right to the sand dune and picked me up. She pushed me right to the water, and once again we all had a good laugh. When she stopped, I got out and walked behind it. It was wonderful to walk on the beach, pushing it to get exercise. It definitely draws attention. It was an awesome help. If you didn't know they exist, as we didn't, take advantage of one if you go to the beach. The beach wheelchairs are funny but enable you to even go to the beach on the sand with many laughs attached.

I decided last summer to buy a three-wheeled bicycle. I believed God's Word to be true and wanted to ride with Dylan. One day after bringing the bike home, Dylan was determined to get me on the bike to ride. I got on it but my feet kept moving off the pedals. God bless Dylan. He told me to hang on. I held the brake to not move down our driveway, which has a small decline down hill; I realized if I let go of the brake, I would end up in the middle of the busy road we live on. Dylan went into our garage and got some duct tape. He duct taped my feet to the pedals so I could ride. I rode down our driveway and back up. It was a big deal for me to ride, even with my feet taped. How we laughed about it that day and still laugh when we think about his little mind using duct tape on my feet.

Just when I thought my scooter crashing days were over, one day, Dylan and I went spring shopping at Kmart. We had to go outside across the parking lot to get mulch for my flower garden. I drove down a ramp to go to the mulch site. On the way back to the store to pay, I drove up the ramp at an angle. Once again, I flipped my scooter. It landed on top of me in the parking lot. Dylan let go of our shopping cart and pulled the scooter off me and pulled me up off the ground. This incident was upsetting, to say the least. I realized I had to drive straight up ramps and not at an angle. God's Word says we are to rejoice in our suffering and that he will not tempt us beyond what we can bear. When you remember God uses every circumstance for our good, these times are bearable. First Corinthians 10:13 states, "No temptation has seized you except what is common to man. And God is faithful; he will not let you be tempted beyond what you can bear. But when you are tempted, he will also provide away out, so you can stand up under it." I was sore and shook up afterward. There again I was on display. Obviously shaken, I had to drive my scooter through the store, dealing with many onlooking shoppers who looked at me with such concern. We made our way to the checkout to pay for the mulch. However, God is so good and saw me through it all. I was able to drive us to get lunch and then drive home. Dylan and I now laugh about crashing at Kmart.

In 2006, my friend Susan and I attended a Joyce Meyer conference about four hours from our home. The first evening Susan and I attended the conference, the weather was sunny and clear when we entered the conference center. As we left, the weather was very stormy with rain and severe lightning. We had no umbrellas and hurried to find my car, getting soaked in the process. I was on my scooter, and Susan had shoes on with a heel. We looked where we thought we parked my car, but it took some time to locate my Honda CRV. There were ten thousand people at the conference. You can imagine how many cars were in the arena's parking lot. Finally, I thought I spotted my car, so Susan unlocked the doors, and I proceeded to get in the car while she drove my scooter to the back of the car to put the scooter in. You know you have a true friend when she will drive your scooter in the pouring rain to put it away, lifting it up to the car without any assistance. As Susan was walking around the car to get in, five ladies approached the car saying, "Hey, that is our car." We both did not believe them as we were relieved to finally get out of the storm. As I sat in the car, I thought it smelled like smoke, and I was thinking, *Someone smoked in my car while we were in the conference.* Susan argued that the car was ours, and one of the ladies said, "Look, my son's college sticker is in the window." We were still not convinced. I asked Susan to look if the rear bumper had duct tape on it. My car was hit in the rear left bumper the weekend before we left, and my dad put duct tape on the sticking out damaged bumper. Susan checked the left bumper, and she shook her head no to me. We could not believe we got in the wrong Honda CRV, which was exactly like mine. How we laughed, and the ladies were kind enough to take us to find our car, which took ten minutes driving around in the rain searching. God has a sense of humor. You may be wondering how we unlocked their car. The ladies were walking to the car at the same time we were. Susan hit the unlock at the same time they did. How bizarre. I guess God was being kind to get us out of rain and lightning while providing a good laugh. When we got back to our motel, we were laughing hysterically to think of how the incident happened. Can you believe the night's laughter wasn't over with the car incident? As we returned to our motel room, we were sitting on the beds laughing about the night. Across from where I was sitting, our clothes were hanging. I looked at the clothes and did not see my black capri pants I brought on the trip. I said to Susan, "I think someone stole my black capri pants. Someone obviously came in here and took my pants." She looked down, and she had on black capri pants. All of a sudden, Susan said, "I thought these were tight on me tonight." We laughed hysterically because she got dressed, grabbing my pair instead of her own. We were overtired and could not believe the happenings of the night.

Remember, it is beneficial to your health to laugh. Rather than making your time waiting on the Lord negative, turn the time around for God's glory; praise him that you are enabled to go and make fun memories during the wait. You will make memories that will last a lifetime. I in no way mean to leave the impression that I am not sad at times and sometimes very sore. However, I choose to trust God, enjoying the journey as I wait on God's promises; I am making a choice to believe and laugh when life throws me curveballs.

Recently, I had a funny incident happen at the ATM machine at the bank where I do my banking. After church one Sunday, Dylan and I went to the ATM to withdraw some money. I input all my information, and the money popped out. I tried reaching the money, but I hesitated with my left hand as I dislocated my pinky finger on that hand and did not want to take a chance of dropping the money on the ground. I asked Dylan to get out of the car to grab the cash. By the time he got around the car to the ATM machine, the money was gone. We could not figure where it went. I proceeded to take more money out, as I still needed cash. This time, Dylan waited for the money to come out and grabbed it quick. My receipt showed I received the first and second withdrawal, however, the first withdrawal disappeared.

I was telling my cousin the story and she laughed so hard, knowing after so many seconds, the machine takes the money back for security reasons. I called the bank the next day, and they did not show the proper credit back to my account. I had to wait three days for the bank to physically count the money in the ATM to see if they were over. Guess what? The bank was over by the exact amount. My cousin and I still laugh about it today. She says she heard it happens but never knew anyone it had happened to. Be quick when getting money from an ATM because the machine might take it back in if you take your time!

One day, I had to pick Dylan up from school because we had a doctor's appointment. My car was parked very close to the ramp in my garage that allows me to take my scooter in and out of the house. As I normally do, I used my scooter to go to my car and get in so I could pick up Dylan. As I opened my door, I had difficulty getting in the driver's seat. I finally landed on my seat, but when I pulled my legs in the car, I lost my left sneaker. The sneaker got stuck between the ramp and the car. It fell down to the garage floor, too low for me to reach and retrieve. I knew I had to leave to pick up Dylan at school. I decided to leave with one shoe on and the other at home in the garage. It was January, and we had snow on the ground. When I picked up Dylan, I was laughing, and he wanted to know what was so funny. I showed him my foot with just a sock on. He was embarrassed. My doctor was so understanding, telling me that some of her patients wear their pajamas and robes to their appointments. My one friend called me Cinderella in the snow. Just another laugh for my history book on laughter.

"A cheerful heart is good medicine" (Proverbs 17:22).

The Way to a Victorious Life

Do you want to live a victorious life? Jesus is the only answer. I have lived both ways—in the world doing it all on my own and as a Christian with God at the helm of my life. In 1996, I asked Jesus to come into my heart and take over. I am so thankful I did.

For the believer, God is our unseen pilot. He guides us and steers our lives. Though we will have trials and tribulations, God is in control. Regardless of what you are going through as a Christian, we have the favoritism of God as his chosen people. As I wait for the manifestation of my healing, I have experienced a personal, powerful, passionate revelation of who God is, and you can have the same awesome opportunity and privilege to know him this way. I have had many ups and downs during this illness, but I would not want to go through one day without God. Though the wait can be difficult, I would never trade knowing personally a loving God who will never let me go. "Never will I leave you, never will I forsake you" (Hebrews 13:5).

What happens to the Christian is orchestrated by God for our benefit. Refuse to quit. If you search the Bible, nothing came overnight for Abraham, Moses, Noah, David, Joseph, etc. These are a few examples. Faith has the ability to stay the course even when your circumstances seem hard and do not yet line up with the Word of God. See Habbakuk 2:3–4, which states, "For the revelation awaits an appointed time; it speaks to an end and will not prove false. Though it linger, wait for it; it will certainly come and will not delay."

We must persevere. The Lord stretches our faith. In Romans 5:5, we also rejoice in our sufferings because we know that suffering produces perseverance; perseverance, character; and character, hope. Although the Lord has stretched my faith, I continue believing his promises knowing all things work together for good to those who love him and are called according to his purpose (read Romans 8:28). I often remind myself and God what his Word says that in all things God works for the good.

As I go to church on my scooter, I will often be asked how I am doing. My response is being thankful for what I have not what I don't yet have. I say, "I am blessed. I thank God I am breathing and my heart is beating. I can see. I can hear. I am alive and have no complaints." Being thankful is a key to enduring the wait. We sing a song at church, "I walk by faith, each step by faith, to live by faith. I put my trust in you." This song has such meaning to me because

I no longer am able to walk, and when I could, I literally would take every step by faith. Appreciate every step if you are able to walk. Never take the simple things in life for granted. You never know when you may lose the ability.

I have been in the fire (sickness) now for nine years. I do not grumble, however. I have struggled with the thief called time. Time is a great enemy to the believer. At the beginning of my disability, it was easier to say God's Word to my situation. As time lingers and things seem tougher, I wonder, "When, God, when? And why, God, why?" These questions are normal; however, you and I need to remember God is making us into what he wants us to be. He will restore us when the time is perfect. From the time our son was in second grade to today, when he is in eleventh grade, I believe each year is the time that I will walk unassisted. I keep believing God and await that glorious day when I see what he has been preparing me for.

Expect the favor of the Lord in the fire. The fire will not harm the child of God; Jesus gets close to you when the fire is burning. Don't let the fire (whatever trial you may be dealing with) scare you. God will do a great work in the fire (cleansing and purifying you) to make you all he created you for. When you come out, you and I will be purified as gold.

Remember to stay positive through the fire. God is with you in the fire if you belong to him. It is never hopeless with Jesus. Build your life in Christ, and you will not be blown away by storms you face. If you fix your eyes on Jesus, the storms of life will not erase your smile. There may be times when it will seems that others are being blessed while you struggle, but keep looking up. The attitude of your faith needs to refuse to be driven back by circumstances.

Do not compare yourself with people of this world. Carnal comparison is an urgent danger to the child of God. Also, comparing with Christian friends is just as bad. You may think, *Why don't they have the struggles I have?"* We all have struggles, just not the same ones. Remember everything may look fine with another person. However, you never know someone else's life until you climb into it. An example is Dylan wanted a new friend to come over to our house, but he was concerned what this friend would think about his dad not living here. It turned out the friend's mom had a boyfriend, and his parents were soon getting divorced. Dylan's eyes were opened to the fact that a lot of people have issues unknown to us, so it's best to not compare. Keep your eyes on eternity and do not lose sight of Jesus. Your faith will become depleted when your eye is off your only source (Jesus). God is faithful. Hang on during the hard times. Remember how powerful words are to our circumstances. In Numbers 14:28, God tells us about what we speak: "As surely as I live, declares the Lord, I will do to you the very things I heard you say." Take God at his Word. There is power in confessing his Word out loud.

To receive, you must believe that what you ask for in prayer is granted to you. I used to think my receiver was broken until I realized I only had to believe I receive before I actually receive the manifestation. Just as you would take your shot or medicine or pill each day, we must take God's medicine daily also. God's medicine is his Word. I have included healing scriptures in the last chapter of this book.

I try to read a page daily as my medicine. It is important to get scriptures into your spirit, as healing comes from the inside out. Healing begins on the inside before you ever see it on the outside. Continually claim your healing and the promises of God. When others see symptoms and do not understand the hope in you, keep walking and speaking in faith, knowing God's Word will not return unto him void (Isaiah 55:11). You will see and feel the manifestation in your body. Your body will line up with the Word of God. Jeremiah 1:12 states, "You have seen correctly, for I am watching to see that my Word is fulfilled."

Praise brings breakthrough. Thank the Lord for your healing even when you don't feel it in your body or feel like doing it. I know firsthand that it is difficult when you are not feeling well, but thank God anyway for your breakthrough. I have been down a very long road and came to realize you cannot go by how you are feeling. It is not about how you feel but who you know—Jesus Christ, our Savior. Remember the God kind of faith "calls things that are not as though they were" (Romans 4:17). In other words, those things that are not yet seen but do in fact exist in the spirit. Faith is not the denial of problems, but the denial of their right to exist in a believer's body in light of God's promises. An example of faith does not deny that a sickness exists, but it denies the right of that sickness to exist in a believer's body because of the promise of healing found in God's Word. I was in denial for a long time. In the past, if someone asked me what is wrong with me I would respond, "I fell walking into work and hurt my back." I would never say that I have MS. I didn't want to claim the disease and lived in fear that somehow MS would get worse by talking about it. Thank God I have changed now. I am not afraid to say MS, knowing Jesus is my healer. I recently met a man at my chiropractic appointment who came out to my car while I was getting ready to leave and said to me, "I just found out we were diagnosed with the same thing." He could not or would not say MS. I found it strange but then realized he was where I used to be, and he was unable to admit the truth. I do not believe we need to speak constantly claiming the disease, but I have learned telling the truth will not stop our awesome God from moving in his timing. A friend of mine told me a story that I shared with the man at my chiropractic appointment. Jesus already paid the price for you and me. You would not go to a store and pay a bill that was already paid for you. The same is true for healing. Jesus already paid the price. Let his will be done as you are changed by the experience. God's definition of faith is found in Hebrews 11:1: "Faith is being sure of what we hope for, and certain of what we do not see." The formula for faith is believing in your heart and speaking out of your mouth.

I know most of the books on sickness available are learning to cope with the disease. However, I pray you find this book to be the only way to live a victorious life and enjoy your journey as you wait for God to move in your life. God wants us walking in his will for our lives and to be whole. Remember Jesus said in Matthew 19:26, "With men this is impossible, but all things are possible with God" (AMP). It does take discipline, but it is well worth it. Your life will be miraculously changed, and you will never want to go back to your old way of life. God loves each of you.

Keep smiling. With God in control, you have everything to smile about. "For I know the plans I have for you; declares the Lord, plans to prosper you and not to harm you, plans to give you hope and a future" (Jeremiah 29:11). Remember, it is not a matter of the promise; it is just a matter of the time. If God said it in his Word, it will surely come to pass. In the interim (the waiting time), he will enable you to continue and change you, as he is doing for me. My pastor always reminds us that his eye is on the clock and his hand is on the thermostat, meaning God knows the amount of time we can stand this trial and how much heat we can take.

Roller Coaster to Victory

I used to enjoy roller coaster rides, but after recent happenings in my life, I'm not so sure I do any longer. As I have revealed earlier, my husband and I have been separated for approximately two years at my request because of his abuse of alcohol.

I started realizing how ill Jeff was around December 2007 when our gas and electric company informed me the day after Christmas that they were scheduled to shut our gas and electric off in two days. The bill had not been paid since July. Jeff had always paid (I thought) our utility bill since he moved out. I was shocked that he was not paying any bills other than his motel bill each week.

A month earlier, Dylan and I wanted to celebrate Jeff's birthday with him by having him over for breakfast. Although we were separated, I tried to keep things as normal as possible for Dylan because I loved my husband and held on to the hope he would get the necessary help and move back home so we could be a family again. I did his laundry and would ask him to dinner. Often, he would not come, or if he did, he sat at the table and never ate.

He never came to our home for his birthday. He planned to come over, but an hour later, he called to say he didn't feel good. We ate breakfast without him. We set his gifts aside until he came over four days later. I was upset at Jeff because Dylan made a nice breakfast for his special day. I never realized until later why he couldn't come over and how very sick he was.

Christmas came that year, and Jeff came over in the morning to open gifts. He didn't stay long, and I noticed when he tried to get up out of the chair, he fell back down. His balance seemed off. This was so sad for Dylan and me to see. Dylan helped him to the car with his gifts. We cried after he left.

We didn't see Jeff for four weeks. I had to go one day to get his checkbook to pay bills when I realized he wasn't paying any bills. I knew because he hadn't seen his son for a month something was very wrong. I always tried to talk to him about the fact that he is missing his fourteen-year-old's life and that he needed help for his alcohol addiction. I offered to take him and do whatever to get him well. Jeff was in denial and told me he didn't have a problem. Dylan also tried to tell him we would take him for help.

A month after Christmas, Jeff called me, begging me to let him come home to get better for a couple of days. I kept telling him no, as I physically could not help him. I knew he needed a doctor or hospital. He had been falling, and I could not get him home. Dylan was at a friend's house, and I would have had to go alone. I insisted he needed professional help and offered to take him anywhere. I knew coming home was not the answer.

He was desperate but still did not want to give in. I decided to call his family. Through this ordeal, I was honest with his dad, but he wasn't hearing me and was in denial also. When I called his brother in New Jersey, he acted a bit surprised and was going to call Jeff and ask how he was. Jeff was very good at disguising any problems to his family. His brother seemed to be in denial like his dad, so I decided to call his sister. I had Jeff heavy on my heart, and although I thought his sister would be angry with me because Jeff and I were separated, I knew I had to call her and leave her attitude toward me to God.

When I called her, she was most appreciative and extremely concerned about her brother. We talked, and I told her now sick he was and asked her opinion on what I should do.

Carol (his sister) decided she was going to call him and tell him he had to go to the hospital. She called Jeff, and at first he said, "I'll see how I feel and maybe I'll go tomorrow." She told him he needed to go and get help today (Sunday). Carol told him she would call the ambulance and meet him at his motel to follow the ambulance to the hospital. Unsure what he should do, Jeff called me. After we talked, I encouraged him he needed to get help. Jeff told me he was undecided but that he might as well go. I believe he knew how sick he was and he had better get help. I called his sister to ask her to call the ambulance.

By now it was 6:00 p.m. on Sunday. I told Carol I would meet them at the hospital. I called my parents and asked them to take me. They came right down. Dylan did not want to go. He stayed with some neighbors. He did not have school the next day, so he spent the night, as I returned home quite late.

When I arrived with my parents at the hospital, Jeff and his sister and her husband were there. I went to where Jeff, was and he looked yellow (jaundice). The doctor in the ER ran a series of tests, and we awaited the results. Some time had passed when I decided to go ask the doctor if any results were in.

He came in to Jeff's ER cubicle and said, "Yes, the test results are in." I had to say, "Well, what are they"? His bedside manner was left behind at doctor school.

He told us (Jeff included) that he had cirrhosis of the liver in its final stage. Jeff asked if he could have a liver transplant. The doctor told him he would have to wait six months to be strong enough for surgery. I asked about alcohol rehabilitation. The hospital I chose to have the ambulance take him to had a rehab program; however, the doctor told us that he was too sick and could not handle rehab. The doctor also told Jeff that he could die that night. His liver was not functioning.

I believed God's Word to me five years earlier that Jeff would not die. I think that is what sustained Dylan and me through the coming weeks. Jeff did not want to die. He kept telling me, and I tried to be positive, even telling him about the Lord's Word to me. He became very humble and wanted his Bible and my pastor to come to see him. Jeff was put in the intensive care unit.

During the time that Jeff was hospitalized, I was so

thankful that he finally was going to get the help he so badly needed. Jeff was in ICU for one week and then transferred to a regular hospital room. Jeff had no health insurance, so he did not qualify for a private room. He had roommates throughout his stay. The first week Jeff was in a regular room, we met with our attorney. Jeff and I already had a will, but our attorney prepared a health care proxy, a living will, a power of attorney, and added my name to the deed of our business. It is so important to have all this paperwork completed before you or your loved one becomes seriously ill. I was thankful our attorney came to Jeff's hospital room for Jeff to sign what was needed.

Over the next two weeks, Jeff seemed to improve slightly. His social worker even talked about transferring him to a nursing home so he could get stronger.

Something changed about four weeks after he was admitted. Jeff was not eating without being fed. He ate very little and got out of bed only once to sit in a wheelchair. Dylan and I would visit when we could. Dylan was frustrated because we visited every Saturday. I would go with my parents at times and let Dylan stay with friends.

How it bothered me that I could not physically visit him without assistance. I always had to go with someone who could handle my scooter and assist me. I never wanted to use my scooter to visit Jeff but had to remember God uses me to reach others on the scooter. The stress was affecting me, and I lost weight dealing with all the emotion. I believed Jeff would get better and move home.

Jeff's sister had cleaned out his motel room and brought all his belongings to our home. I had boxes of his stuff to sort through as time permitted. Life was definitely turned upside down. Not to mention I had bills that were Jeff's to pay. Jeff and I always had our money separate. I guess it was because he was a bachelor for so long before our marriage. I got used to our financial arrangement, but suddenly it was all in my lap.

Jeff's mind seemed so confused these weeks. I called him often. One day, he wanted me to come get him and take him for a ride. I told him he could not leave the hospital. Another day, he just wanted me to drive by the hospital so he could look out the window and see me. Dylan was due to get off the bus from school, and I explained I didn't have enough time. The hospital was twenty minutes from our home. He did not understand why I couldn't go by the hospital before Dylan arrived home. I kept telling Jeff, "I love you, and we will be down later."

I also had doctors calling me, as I was not always at the hospital, and he was beginning to grow worse. His kidneys were failing, and I had to make the decision not to have the hospital perform dialysis. I knew the liver was the primary problem, and I did not feel he could tolerate kidney dialysis.

That same week, Jeff was asleep during one of our visits. I noticed in his urine bag what looked like bile. I held on to God's Word to me five years prior that Jeff would not die. I had a dear friend and also my pastor who visited Jeff often and prayed for him. Jeff was very receptive to the Word and Jesus in his desperation. I was thankful he even asked for his Bible when he moved into a room.

It was a Thursday, March 6, when one of Jeff's doctors

called and told me he was not good. I called my Pastor, hysterically crying, and asked him if he could go pray for Jeff. I knew Dylan and I were going that night after school. My parents came and took us there to see Jeff. When we arrived at the hospital, Jeff was thrashing his head back and forth; he was on morphine, his eyes were closed, and he was out of it. Dylan left the room with my dad. My mom and I stayed with Jeff. She tried to tell him Karen and Dylan were there. He opened his eyes for a second but went back to what seemed like sleep. I used anointing oil and prayed for Jeff. I asked God that he would not suffer any longer. I prayed for God's will and to take him home to heaven if it was God's time. Dylan went in after I left and told his dad he loved him. He opened his eyes briefly and went back to sleep. We left the hospital.

We came home and I called a prayer chain for a phone counselor to stand in agreement with me for a new liver and his total healing. I still believed as I went to bed that he would not die.

I took the phone to bed, which I normally never did, and tried to sleep. At 2:00 a.m., my phone rang. I saw Saint Joseph's Hospital on caller ID. It was the hospital chaplain, who said to me, "You know your husband has recently taken a turn for the worse." I said, "Yes." He said, "I'm sorry. He just passed away." I think I was numb but quickly called Jeff's sister. She told me she would call the funeral director for me. I called my family and Jeff's dad. I did not wake Dylan up. I thought I would tell him when he awoke for school.

When Dylan's alarm went off, I went into his room

and said, "I want to talk to you. Meet me in the living room." He quickly got up, came out to me, and said, "He's gone, isn't he?" I said yes in tears. Dylan fell on the floor and cried. We both cried and agreed we did not want him to suffer any more. Dylan or I could not understand God's Word to me that he would not die. We now know Jeff is in heaven and will live for eternity. I believe that is what God meant when he told me years earlier, "Remember, Jeff will not die." We still both struggled with his death.

Dylan got mad at God. I know he still questions why he lost his father at fourteen years old. He also doubts my healing from multiple sclerosis. He has seen my struggle more than anyone. I tell him God's timing is perfect, and we will see the goodness of the Lord in the land of the living (Psalm 27:13).

Life became most stressful when we had Jeff's funeral. I chose to have private calling hours and a memorial service at the funeral home following. I made the decision for private services because Jeff had three businesses locally over the years, and I could not deal with all the old customers. It seemed he knew everyone, and I was wiped out emotionally with the five weeks, four days he was in the hospital. His family and mine invited family and friends to attend. He was only fifty-four years old, and it was an extremely sad time.

Dylan and I also decided on a closed casket. I tried to persuade Dylan that he may want to see his dad at peace one last time. Dylan was sure he did not want the casket open, so I complied. I am certain Jeff would never want me to upset Dylan, who was his pride and joy. I got resistance from his family, but they knew I had the final say. His family decided to come earlier than Dylan and I, and they had the casket open to view Jeff. It was closed before we arrived.

The memorial service was comforting. My Pastor, who spent time with Jeff over the five weeks in the hospital, spoke of him in heaven and for us to hold on to all the memories. Dylan prayed with a friend of mine the night Jeff died. My friend prayed for Dylan to have peace and to know his dad was okay.

The night of the funeral, Dylan came in my room. He had a weird dream, and he told me about it. We laughed. It was very bizarre. He eventually went back to his room to sleep. When I awoke, I let Dylan sleep, as he was still on leave from school for his dad's death. When he finally got out of bed, he came out in the kitchen where I was, and he said, "Oh, by the way, I saw Dad in my room after my dream last night." I questioned why he didn't mention it in the middle of the night. He told me he didn't want to get into it then.

Dylan went on to tell me when he woke up from his odd dream, his dad was in the corner of his room. I asked, "How did he look?" Dylan said he saw him from the waist up, and he looked healthy, like the old Jeff. Jeff mouthed, "I love you," and off he went through the wall upward. I couldn't believe Dylan really saw Jeff.

As we were talking, my friend that prayed with Dylan the night Jeff died called me. She said, "Karen, God just spoke to me and told me he gave Dylan the vision of Jeff you prayed for, and Dylan's going to be fine." God knew I would think Dylan had a dream of his dad. God's Word was confirmed and showed me and Dylan that Jeff was okay. Dylan had peace about his Dad's death after his vision that night. Dylan will never stop missing his dad, but rests, knowing Jeff is with the Lord, and one day we will join him in eternity.

I want to tell you the victory is that Jeff went to be with the Lord in heaven. He became very humble and sweet in the hospital. I so wanted and believed he would finally get well and our marriage would be restored. I wasn't worried while he was hospitalized because I was so happy we could begin again minus alcohol. Then he died. I must remember Jeff is well now and alcohol free.

It is hard now Jeff is gone. Our wedding anniversary just passed and to never again celebrate that special day is unbelievably difficult. I know he is at peace; however, the finality to know we will never see or talk to him again on earth is hard.

Life has turned upside down. Jeff had no health insurance. I receive hospital and other medical bills each week. My attorney is negotiating payments, so I am awaiting the finality of doctor and hospital bills. I have to trust God will take care of Dylan and me. Nevertheless, this world and all the stuff, including medical bills, will pass away. I look around our house with many memories that not even one Jeff was able to take with him. Where you go when you die is all that really matters. I am praising God that Jeff is home in heaven. If you are married, appreciate your spouse regardless of his or her failures and faults. You never know when one day he or she will be gone.

God is faithful and will work all these things together for your good (Romans 8:28). I don't want to start over but pray for God's will above my will. I always wanted Jeff to see my healing and finally see what I have believed for so long. I know Jeff will see the manifestation when I see him again in heaven. Until that day, I am trusting God is in control, and his grace is sufficient (2 Corinthians 12:9) and will meet all our needs. Many times I have wanted off this ride, believing it is too painful and difficult. The grace of God is the only thing that has sustained me through the ups and downs of this roller coaster called life.

May God richly bless you as you walk in faith and wait to see the manifestation of your healing. Don't look to a man for your healing. As you grow in your relationship with the Lord, something will be kicking on the inside of you to push ahead when you want to quit and give up. Never give up.

To begin your healing journey, you must put Jesus at the helm of your life by asking Jesus into your heart. God wants you healed more than you do. He provided the way by dying on the cross for our sins and took all sickness with him on the cross also. A wonderful movie to watch on video is *The Passion of the Christ*. You will see the suffering that Christ endured for us on the cross for our sins and sicknesses.

If you want to spend eternity in heaven and walk healed and whole, you just need to say a simple prayer and receive what he has already done by faith. Say the following prayer if you have not already done so.

Salvation Prayer

Heavenly Father, I come to you in the name of Jesus. Your Word says, "Whosoever shall call on the name of the Lord shall be saved" (Acts 2:21, KJV). I am calling on you. I pray and ask Jesus to come into my heart and take over. I cannot do this alone any longer. I repent of all my sins, and I believe in my heart that Jesus is Lord, died on the cross, and that God raised him from the dead. I give you my life in Jesus's name.

Healing Scriptures

I have included healing scriptures from the Word of God. Speak them out of your mouth daily, and you will find they will become more real to you than your sickness or any symptom. Your body will line up with the Word of God.

Say the following scriptures out loud daily. Charles Capps said in his book, *God's Creative Power for Healing*, "To be spoken by mouth three times a day until faith comes, then once a day to maintain faith. If circumstances grow worse, double the dosage. There are no harmful side effects."

I firmly believe with Jesus as your Lord, by taking proper care of your body and a positive attitude, you will have optimal health.

> If you listen carefully to the voice of the Lord your God, and do what is right in his eyes, if you pay attention to his commands and keep all his decrees, I will not bring on you any of the diseases I brought on the Egyptians, for I am the Lord, who heals you.
>
> Exodus 15:26

Worship the Lord your God and his blessing will be on your food and water. I will take away sickness from among you.

Exodus 23:25

You will be blessed more than any other people; none of your men or women will be childless nor any of your livestock without young. The Lord will keep you free from every disease. He will not inflict on you the horrible diseases you knew in Egypt, but will inflict them on all who hate you.

Deuteronomy 7:14–15

Not one of all the Lord's good promises failed; every one was fulfilled.

Joshua 21:45

I have heard your prayer and seen your tears, I will heal you.

2 Kings 20:5

The Lord gives strength to his people; the Lord blesses his people with peace.

Psalm 29:11

O Lord my God, I called to you for help and you healed me.

Psalm 30:2

Who forgives all your sins and heals all your diseases.

Psalm 103:2–3

He sent forth his Word and healed them; he rescued them from the grave.

Psalm 107:20

I will not die but live and will proclaim what the Lord has done.

Psalm 118:17

My son, pay attention to what I say; listen closely to my words. Do not let them out of your sight, keep them within your heart; for they are life to those who find them, and health to a man's whole body.

Proverbs 4:20–22

A cheerful heart is good medicine, but a crushed spirit dries up the bones.

Proverbs 17:22

So do not fear, I am with you; Do not be dismayed, for I am your God. I will strengthen you and help you; I will uphold you with my righteous right hand.

Isaiah 41:10

Surely he took up our infirmities and carried our sorrows, yet we considered him stricken by God, smitten by him, and afflicted. But he was pierced for our transgressions, he was crushed for our iniquities; the punishment that brought us peace was upon him, and by his wounds we are healed.

Isaiah 53:4–5

The Lord said to me, "You have seen correctly, for I am watching to see that my Word is fulfilled."

Jeremiah 1:12

Heal me, O Lord, and I will be healed; save me and I will be saved, for you are the one I praise.

Jeremiah 17:14

For I know the plans I have for you, declares the Lord, plans to prosper you and not to harm you, plans to give you hope and a future. Then you will call upon me and come and pray to me, and I will listen to you. You will seek me and find me with all your heart. I will be found by you, declares the Lord, and will bring you back from captivity.

Jeremiah 29:11–14

"But I will restore you to health and heal your wounds," declares the Lord.

Jeremiah 30:17

I will heal my people and let them enjoy abundant peace and security.

Jeremiah 33:6

Let the weakling say, "I am strong."

Joel 3:10

When the evening came, many who were demon possessed were brought to him and he drove out the spirits with a word and healed all the sick. This was to fulfill what was spoken through the prophet Isaiah: He took up our infirmities and carried our diseases.

Matthew 8:16–17

Have faith in God, Jesus answered. I tell you the truth, if anyone says to this mountain, "Go throw yourself into the sea" and does not doubt in his heart but believes that what he says will happen, it will be done for him. Therefore, I tell you whatever you ask for in prayer believe that you have received it, and it will be yours.

Mark 11:22–24

The people all tried to touch him, because power was coming from him and healing them all.

Luke 6:19

Crowds gathered also from the towns around Jerusalem, bringing their sick and those tormented by evil spirits, and all of them were healed.

Acts 5:16

How God anointed Jesus of Nazareth with the Holy Spirit and power, and how he went around doing good and healing all who were under the power of the devil, because God was with them.

Acts 10:38

Therefore, the promise comes by faith, so that it may be by grace and may be guaranteed to all Abraham's offspring—not only to those who are of the law but also to those who are of the faith of Abraham. He is the father of us all. As it is written: "I have made you a father of many nations." He is our father in the sight of God, in whom he believed—the God who gives life to the dead and calls things that are not as though they were. Against all hope, Abraham in hope believed and so became the father of many nations, just as it had been said to him, so shall your offspring be. Without weakening in his faith, he faced the fact that his body was as good as dead—since he was about a hundred years old and that Sarah's womb was also dead. Yet he did not waiver through unbelief regarding the promise of God but was strengthened in his faith and gave glory to God, being fully persuaded that God had power to do what he had promised."

Romans 4:16–21

And if the spirit of him who raised Jesus from the dead is living in you, he who raised Christ from the dead will also give life to your mortal bodies through his spirit, who lives in you.

Romans 8:11

As it is written, "How beautiful are the feet of those who bring good news!"

Romans 10:15

Be joyful in hope, patient in affliction, faithful in prayer.

Romans 12:12

May the God of hope fill you with all joy and peace as you trust in him, so that you may overflow with hope by the power of the Holy Spirit.

Romans 15:13

Christ redeemed us from the curse of the law by becoming a curse for us, for it is written: cursed is everyone who is hung on a tree.

Galatians 3:13

For it is God who works in you to will and to act according to his good purpose.

Philippians 2:13

Let us hold unswervingly to the hope we profess, for he who promised is faithful.

Hebrews 10:23

So do not throw away your confidence, it will be richly rewarded. You need to persevere so that when you have done the will of God, you will receive what he has promised.

Hebrews 10:36

Jesus Christ is the same yesterday and today and forever.

Hebrews 13:8

Submit yourselves then, to God. Resist the devil, and he will flee from you. Come near to God and he will come near to you.

James 4:7–8

He himself bore our sins in his body on the tree, so that we might die to sins and live for righteousness; by his wounds, you have been healed.

1 Peter 2:24

Dear friends, if our hearts do not condemn us, we have confidence before God and receive from him anything we ask because we obey his commands and do what pleases him.

1 John 3:21–22

This is the confidence we have in approaching God: that if we ask anything according to his will, he hears us. And if we know that he hears us—whatever we ask—we know that we have what we asked of him.

1 John 5:14–15

Dear friend, I pray that you may enjoy good health and that all may go well with you even as you soul is getting along well.

3 John 2

Final Note

I began writing on November 15, 2001, and saw a note I wrote that my son Dylan told me I had to include. He told me this on November 20, 2001.

Dylan said, "Mom, when you finish your book, you should put "Jesus healed me." Praise God. What wisdom my eight-year-old had! By faith, the Lord has changed my life totally for the good, and healing will be the reward. Thank you to Dylan for standing by me through thick and thin. At such a young age, Dylan was calling those things that were not as though they were. Dylan said what God says about me. God is faithful. To have faith is to believe in the faithfulness of God. In Psalm 145:13 God says, "The Lord is faithful to all his promises and loving toward all he has made." To God be the glory.

*Drawn by Dylan when he was 5 years old. Karen
planned to include it when she finished her book*

In Loving Memory

Jeffrey L. Walther
November 24, 1953–March 7, 2008

It's a miracle you made it to heaven.
You left me here to fend alone.
We have a beautiful boy who is almost full grown.
We miss your presence but know you are with God.
Our life's story must still be told.
The Lord will never leave us and
see us through each day.
Pray we can endure this journey
no matter what comes our way.
We thank God you are with him.
Until we meet again, know how much we love you.
You are free from the pain and your addiction.
Life has just begun for eternity for you, my dear.
Remember in my heart you will always be near.

Bibliography

McCollum, Edward. "The Story of Protein".

Keith, Velma J. and Monteen Gordon. The How To Herb Book. Pleasant Grove, Utah: Mayfield Publications, 1984.

Haas, Elson M. M.D. Staying Healthy With Nutrition. Berkeley, California: Celestial Arts Publishing, 1992.

Life Extension Online References for Health Concerns http:// www.lef.org/protocols /prtc/-077b.shtml

Embry, Ashton, F. "Vitamin D Supplementation in the Fight Against Multiple Sclerosis". http://www.direct-ms.org/vitamin-d.html

Colbert, Don M.D. "The Most Important Nutrient for the Body." Joyce Meyer Ministries Magazine August 2003.

Liquid Candy: How Soft Drinks Are Harming Americans Health http://www.cspinet.org/sodapop/highlights.htm

Mercola, Joseph Dr. "Each Daily Soda Increases Obesity Risk 60%" 25 February 2001. http://www.mercola.com/2001/feb/28/obesity soft drinks.htm

Anderson, Ross, N.D. Are You Clear of Parasites. http://home.online.no/-sostuve/anderson.html

Holistic Health Solutions: http:www.holistichelp.net/candida.html

Scripture References–NIV Bible (unless otherwise noted)